This Journal
BELONGS TO

_____

_____

DEDICATION

This Body Measurement Tracker book is dedicated to all the hard working, organized people out there who want to keep track of their body measurements.

Your are my inspiration for producing books and I'm honored to be a part of keeping all your body measurement notes all in one place.

This Body Measurement Tracker journal notebook will help you record your details, notes and schedules about your body measurements.

Thoughtfully put together with these sections to record:
Date, Chest, Left Arm, Right Arm, Waist, Hips, Left Thigh, Right Thigh, Left Calf, Right Calf, Weight and Notes.

HOW TO USE THIS BOOK

The purpose of this book is to keep all of your lists and notes all in one place. It will help keep you organized.

This Body Measurement Tracker Journal will allow you to accurately document all of your Body measurements, schedule, and details. It's a great way to chart your course through measuring your body.

Here are examples of the prompts for you to fill in and write about yourself in this book:

1. Date
2. Chest
3. Left Arm
4. Right Arm
5. Waist
6. Hips
7. Left Thigh
8. Right Thigh
9. Left Calf
10. Right Calf
11. Weight
12. Notes - Great for writing your food intake, set goals, fat intake, plan, monitoring, emotions, how you feel, etc or whatever you wish to write.

BODY MEASUREMENTS TRACKER

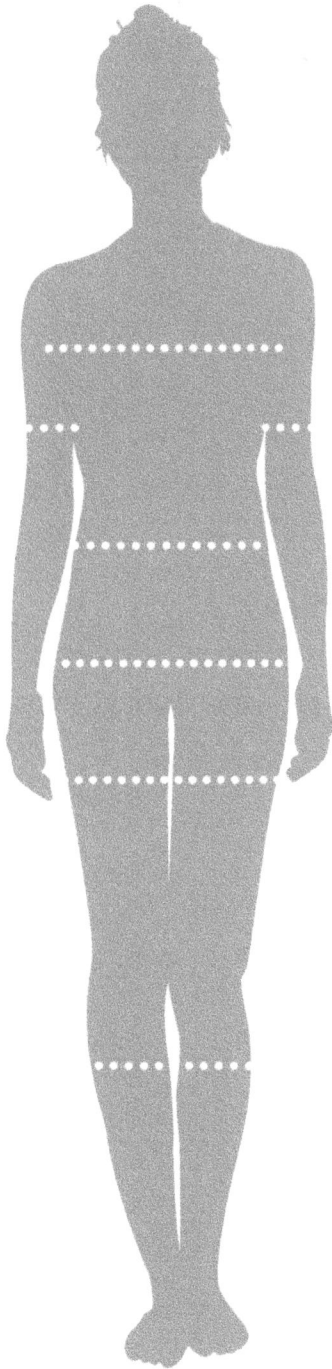

BEFORE

DATE

CHEST

LEFT ARM

RIGHT ARM

WAIST

HIPS

LEFT THIGH

RIGHT THIGH

LEFT CALF

RIGHT CALF

WEIGHT

NOTES

AFTER

DATE

CHEST

LEFT ARM

RIGHT ARM

WAIST

HIPS

LEFT THIGH

LEFT CALF

RIGHT CALF

WEIGHT

BODY MEASUREMENTS TRACKER

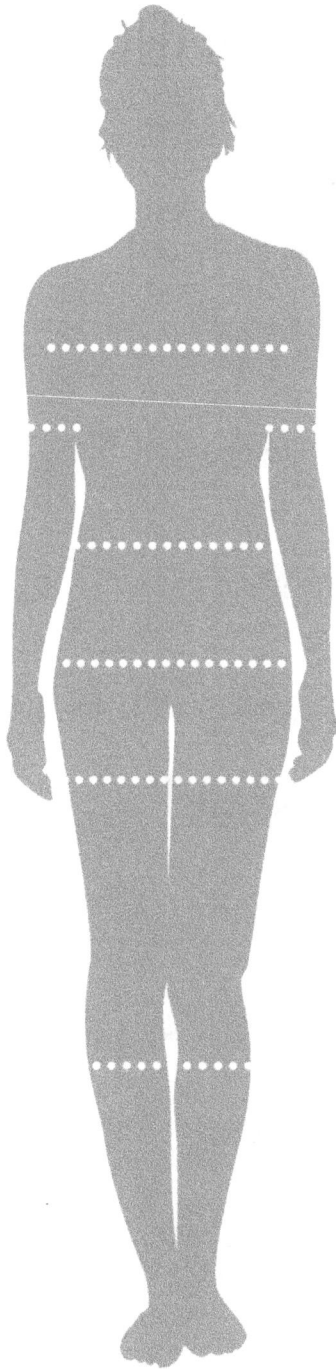

BEFORE

DATE

CHEST

LEFT ARM

RIGHT ARM

WAIST

HIPS

LEFT THIGH

RIGHT THIGH

LEFT CALF

RIGHT CALF

WEIGHT

NOTES

AFTER

DATE

CHEST

LEFT ARM

RIGHT ARM

WAIST

HIPS

LEFT THIGH

LEFT CALF

RIGHT CALF

WEIGHT

BODY MEASUREMENTS TRACKER

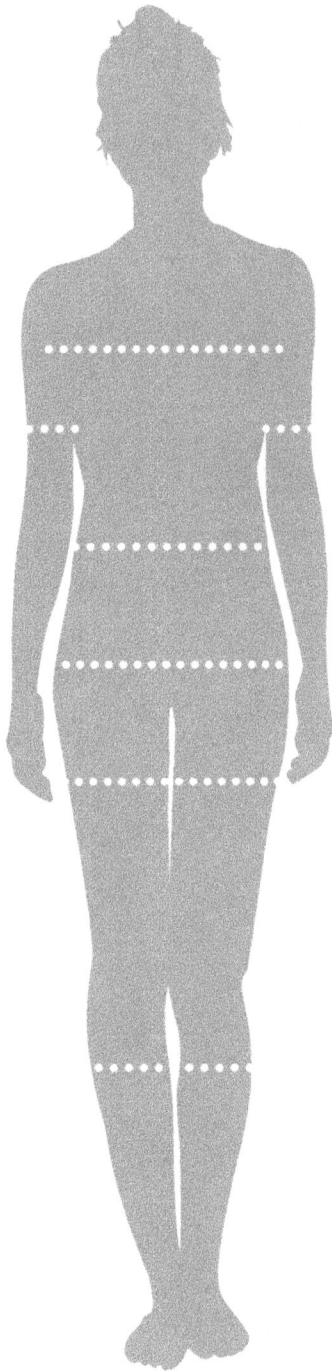

BEFORE

DATE	
CHEST	
LEFT ARM	
RIGHT ARM	
WAIST	
HIPS	
LEFT THIGH	
RIGHT THIGH	
LEFT CALF	
RIGHT CALF	
WEIGHT	

AFTER

DATE	
CHEST	
LEFT ARM	
RIGHT ARM	
WAIST	
HIPS	
LEFT THIGH	
LEFT CALF	
RIGHT CALF	
WEIGHT	

NOTES

BODY MEASUREMENTS TRACKER

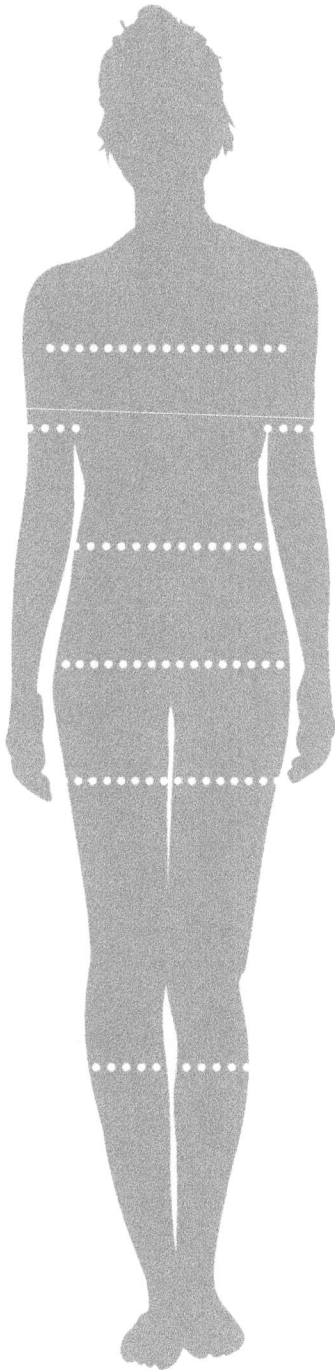

BEFORE

DATE

CHEST

LEFT ARM

RIGHT ARM

WAIST

HIPS

LEFT THIGH

RIGHT THIGH

LEFT CALF

RIGHT CALF

WEIGHT

NOTES

AFTER

DATE

CHEST

LEFT ARM

RIGHT ARM

WAIST

HIPS

LEFT THIGH

LEFT CALF

RIGHT CALF

WEIGHT

BODY MEASUREMENTS TRACKER

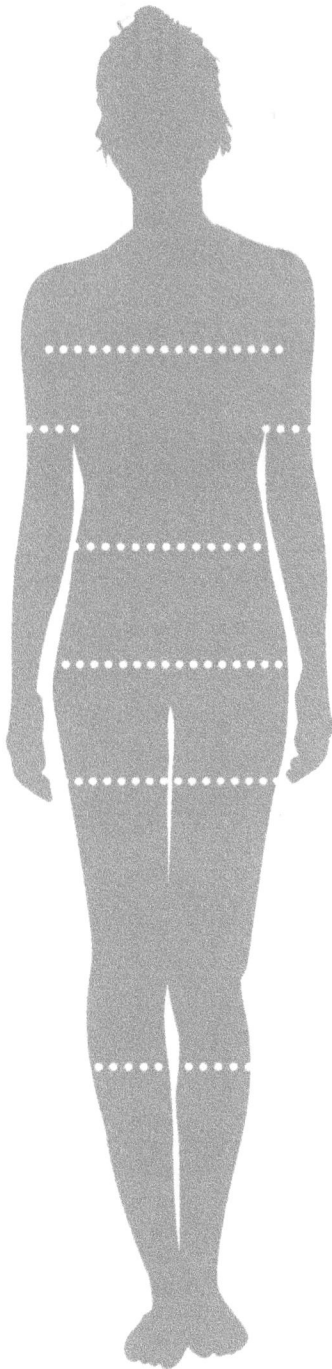

BEFORE

DATE	
CHEST	
LEFT ARM	
RIGHT ARM	
WAIST	
HIPS	
LEFT THIGH	
RIGHT THIGH	
LEFT CALF	
RIGHT CALF	
WEIGHT	

AFTER

DATE	
CHEST	
LEFT ARM	
RIGHT ARM	
WAIST	
HIPS	
LEFT THIGH	
LEFT CALF	
RIGHT CALF	
WEIGHT	

NOTES

BODY MEASUREMENTS TRACKER

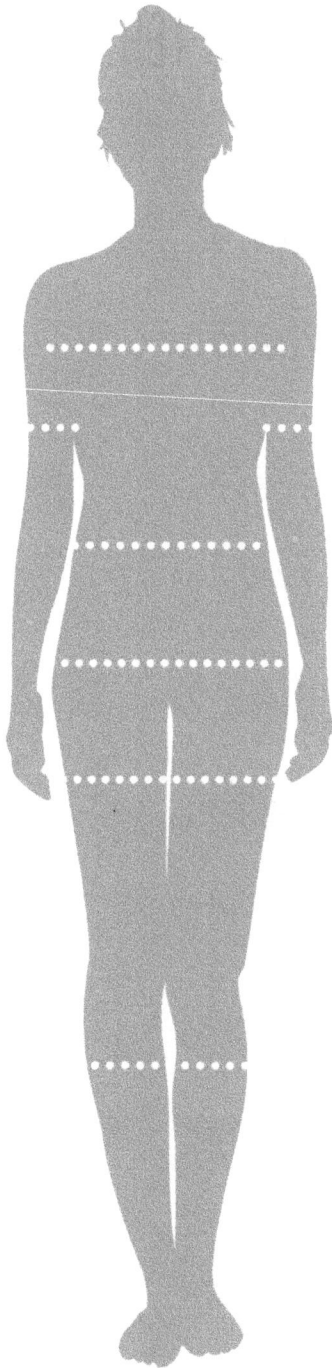

BEFORE

DATE

CHEST

LEFT ARM

RIGHT ARM

WAIST

HIPS

LEFT THIGH

RIGHT THIGH

LEFT CALF

RIGHT CALF

WEIGHT

NOTES

AFTER

DATE

CHEST

LEFT ARM

RIGHT ARM

WAIST

HIPS

LEFT THIGH

LEFT CALF

RIGHT CALF

WEIGHT

BODY MEASUREMENTS TRACKER

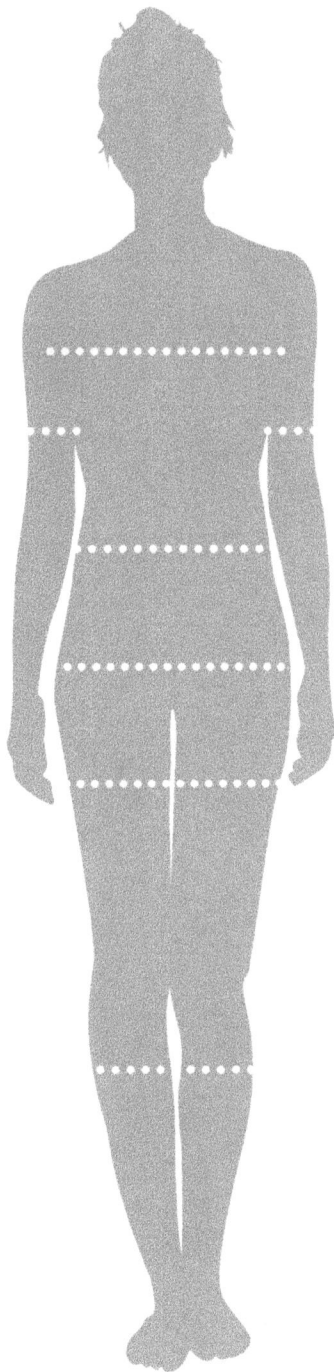

	BEFORE	AFTER
DATE		
CHEST		
LEFT ARM		
RIGHT ARM		
WAIST		
HIPS		
LEFT THIGH		
RIGHT THIGH		
LEFT CALF		
RIGHT CALF		
WEIGHT		

NOTES

BODY MEASUREMENTS TRACKER

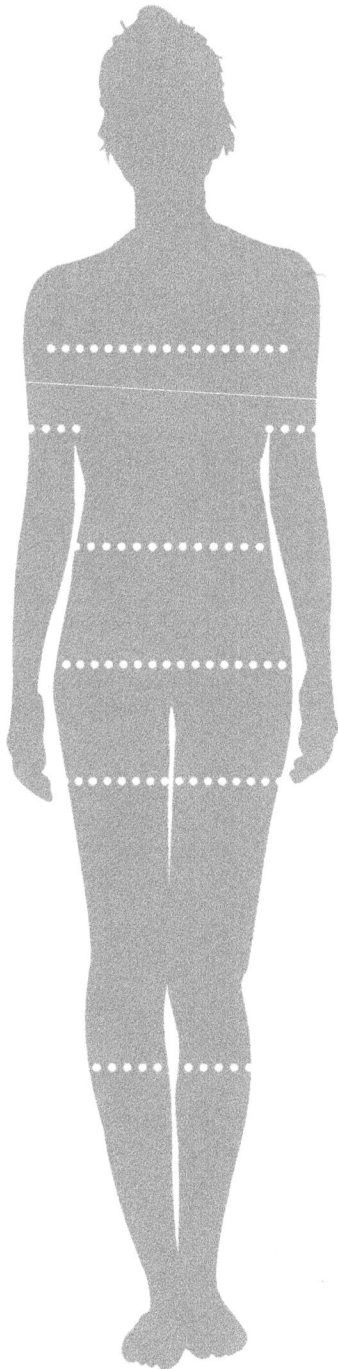

BEFORE

DATE

CHEST

LEFT ARM

RIGHT ARM

WAIST

HIPS

LEFT THIGH

RIGHT THIGH

LEFT CALF

RIGHT CALF

WEIGHT

NOTES

AFTER

DATE

CHEST

LEFT ARM

RIGHT ARM

WAIST

HIPS

LEFT THIGH

LEFT CALF

RIGHT CALF

WEIGHT

BODY MEASUREMENTS TRACKER

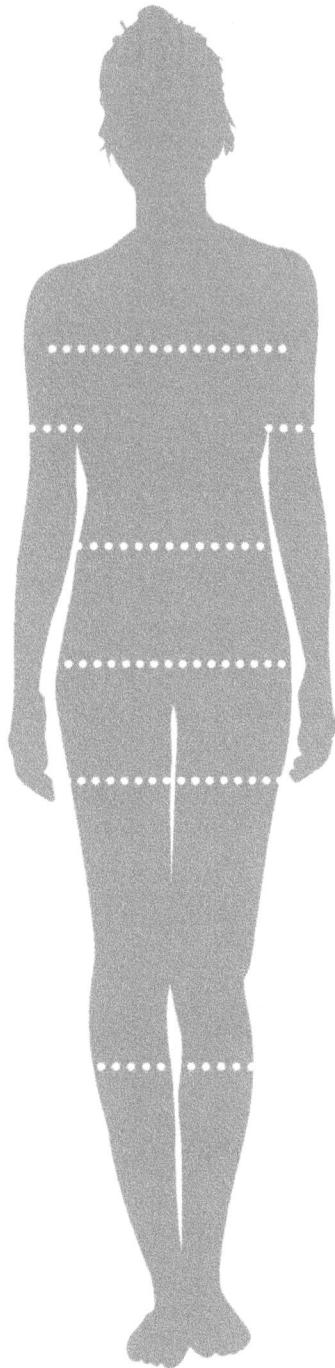

	BEFORE	AFTER
DATE		
CHEST		
LEFT ARM		
RIGHT ARM		
WAIST		
HIPS		
LEFT THIGH		
RIGHT THIGH		
LEFT CALF		
RIGHT CALF		
WEIGHT		
NOTES		

BODY MEASUREMENTS TRACKER

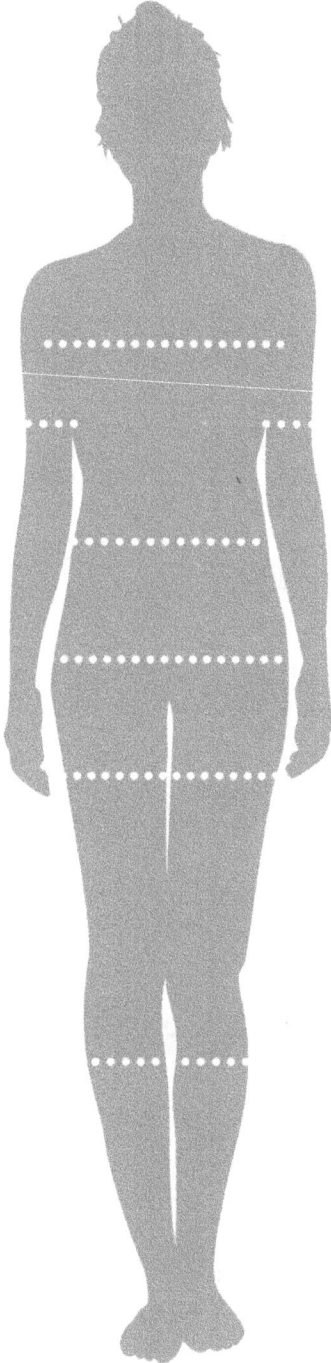

BEFORE

DATE

CHEST

LEFT ARM

RIGHT ARM

WAIST

HIPS

LEFT THIGH

RIGHT THIGH

LEFT CALF

RIGHT CALF

WEIGHT

NOTES

AFTER

DATE

CHEST

LEFT ARM

RIGHT ARM

WAIST

HIPS

LEFT THIGH

LEFT CALF

RIGHT CALF

WEIGHT

BODY MEASUREMENTS TRACKER

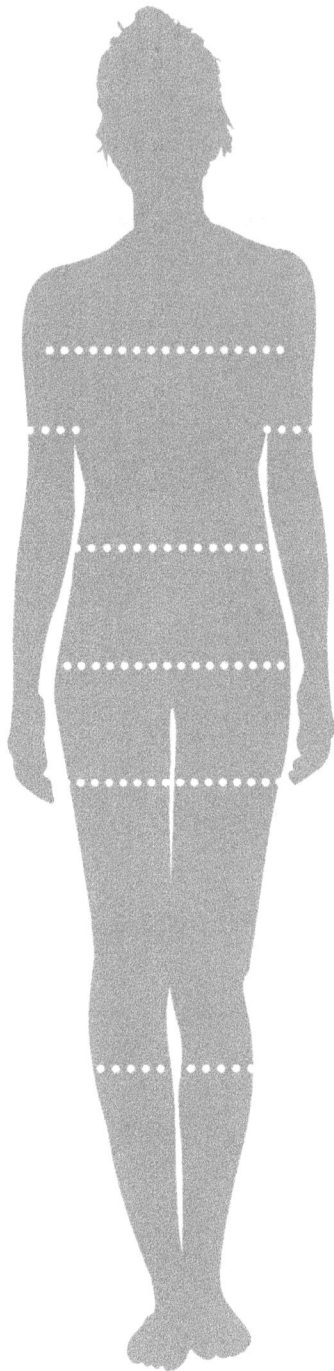

BEFORE

DATE

CHEST

LEFT ARM

RIGHT ARM

WAIST

HIPS

LEFT THIGH

RIGHT THIGH

LEFT CALF

RIGHT CALF

WEIGHT

NOTES

AFTER

DATE

CHEST

LEFT ARM

RIGHT ARM

WAIST

HIPS

LEFT THIGH

LEFT CALF

RIGHT CALF

WEIGHT

BODY MEASUREMENTS TRACKER

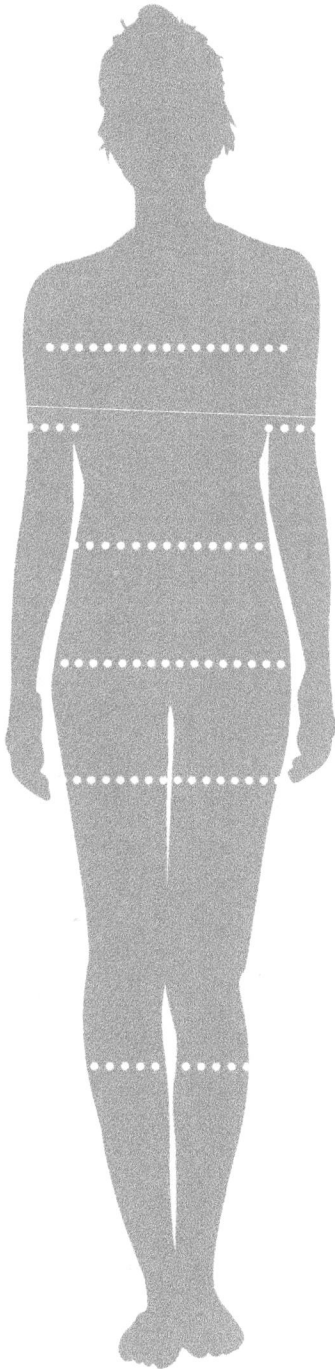

BEFORE

DATE

CHEST

LEFT ARM

RIGHT ARM

WAIST

HIPS

LEFT THIGH

RIGHT THIGH

LEFT CALF

RIGHT CALF

WEIGHT

NOTES

AFTER

DATE

CHEST

LEFT ARM

RIGHT ARM

WAIST

HIPS

LEFT THIGH

LEFT CALF

RIGHT CALF

WEIGHT

BODY MEASUREMENTS TRACKER

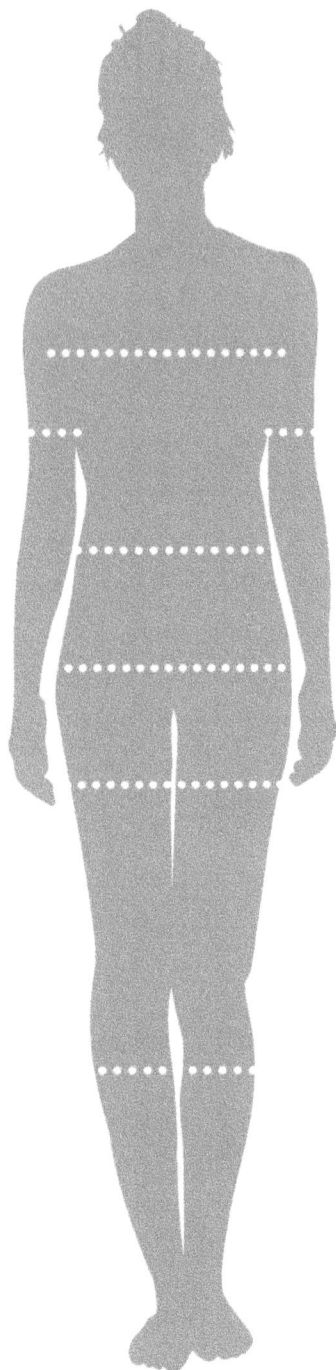

BEFORE

DATE

CHEST

LEFT ARM

RIGHT ARM

WAIST

HIPS

LEFT THIGH

RIGHT THIGH

LEFT CALF

RIGHT CALF

WEIGHT

NOTES

AFTER

DATE

CHEST

LEFT ARM

RIGHT ARM

WAIST

HIPS

LEFT THIGH

LEFT CALF

RIGHT CALF

WEIGHT

BODY MEASUREMENTS TRACKER

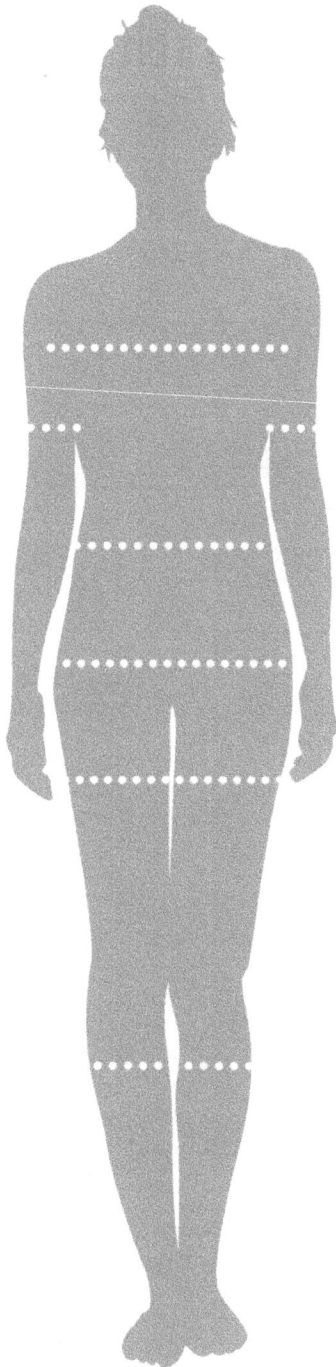

BEFORE

DATE

CHEST

LEFT ARM

RIGHT ARM

WAIST

HIPS

LEFT THIGH

RIGHT THIGH

LEFT CALF

RIGHT CALF

WEIGHT

NOTES

AFTER

DATE

CHEST

LEFT ARM

RIGHT ARM

WAIST

HIPS

LEFT THIGH

LEFT CALF

RIGHT CALF

WEIGHT

BODY MEASUREMENTS TRACKER

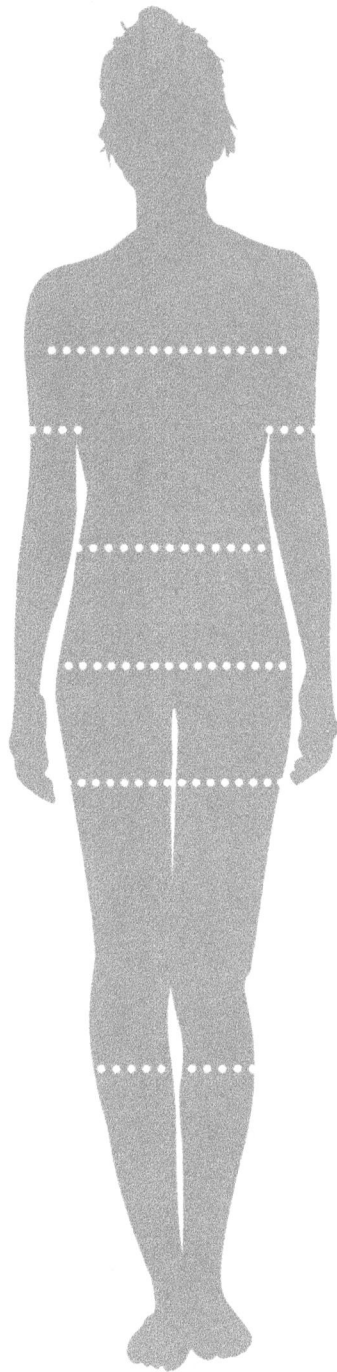

BEFORE

DATE

CHEST

LEFT ARM

RIGHT ARM

WAIST

HIPS

LEFT THIGH

RIGHT THIGH

LEFT CALF

RIGHT CALF

WEIGHT

NOTES

AFTER

DATE

CHEST

LEFT ARM

RIGHT ARM

WAIST

HIPS

LEFT THIGH

LEFT CALF

RIGHT CALF

WEIGHT

BODY MEASUREMENTS TRACKER

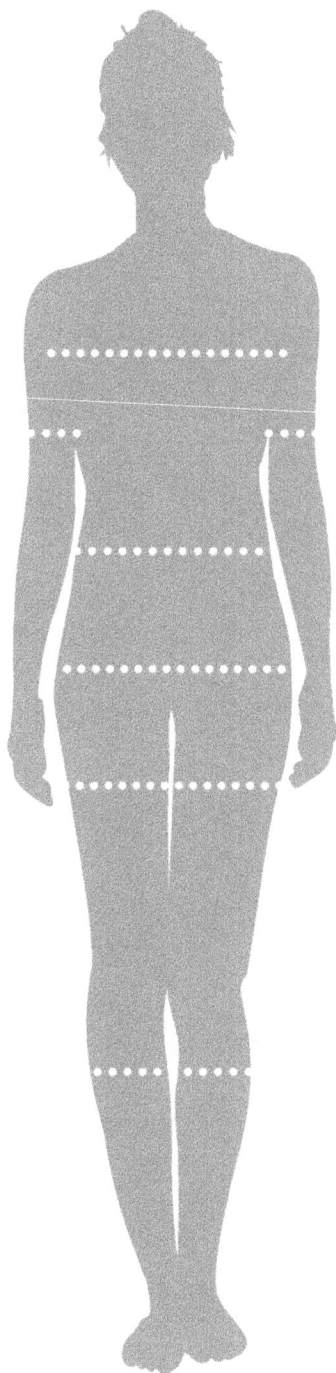

BEFORE

DATE

CHEST

LEFT ARM

RIGHT ARM

WAIST

HIPS

LEFT THIGH

RIGHT THIGH

LEFT CALF

RIGHT CALF

WEIGHT

NOTES

AFTER

DATE

CHEST

LEFT ARM

RIGHT ARM

WAIST

HIPS

LEFT THIGH

LEFT CALF

RIGHT CALF

WEIGHT

BODY MEASUREMENTS TRACKER

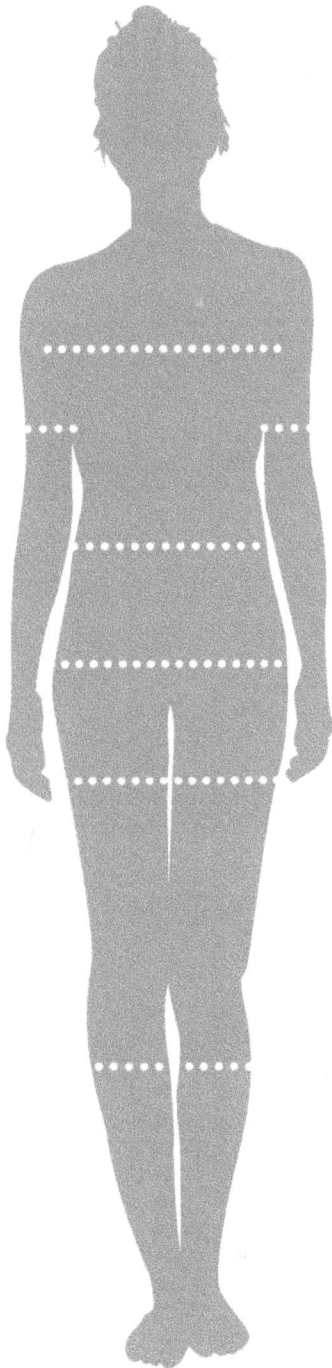

BEFORE

DATE

CHEST

LEFT ARM

RIGHT ARM

WAIST

HIPS

LEFT THIGH

RIGHT THIGH

LEFT CALF

RIGHT CALF

WEIGHT

NOTES

AFTER

DATE

CHEST

LEFT ARM

RIGHT ARM

WAIST

HIPS

LEFT THIGH

LEFT CALF

RIGHT CALF

WEIGHT

BODY MEASUREMENTS TRACKER

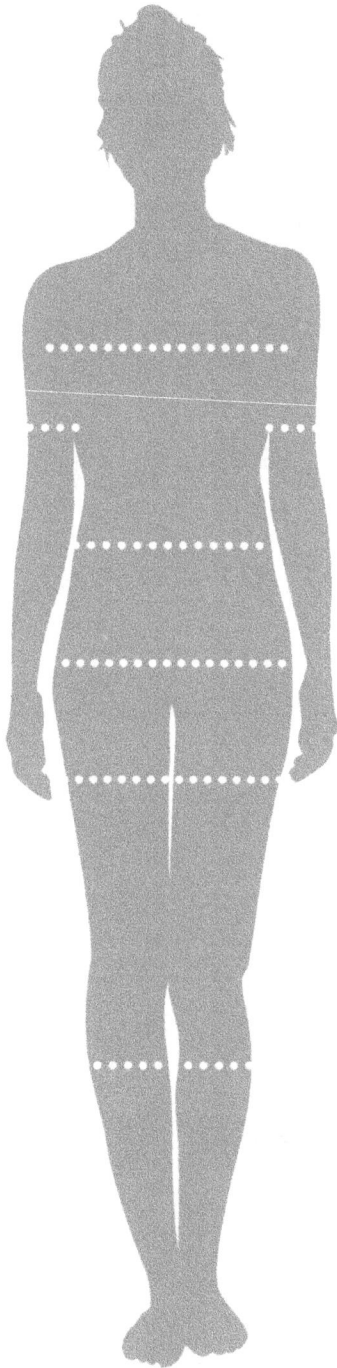

BEFORE

DATE

CHEST

LEFT ARM

RIGHT ARM

WAIST

HIPS

LEFT THIGH

RIGHT THIGH

LEFT CALF

RIGHT CALF

WEIGHT

NOTES

AFTER

DATE

CHEST

LEFT ARM

RIGHT ARM

WAIST

HIPS

LEFT THIGH

LEFT CALF

RIGHT CALF

WEIGHT

BODY MEASUREMENTS TRACKER

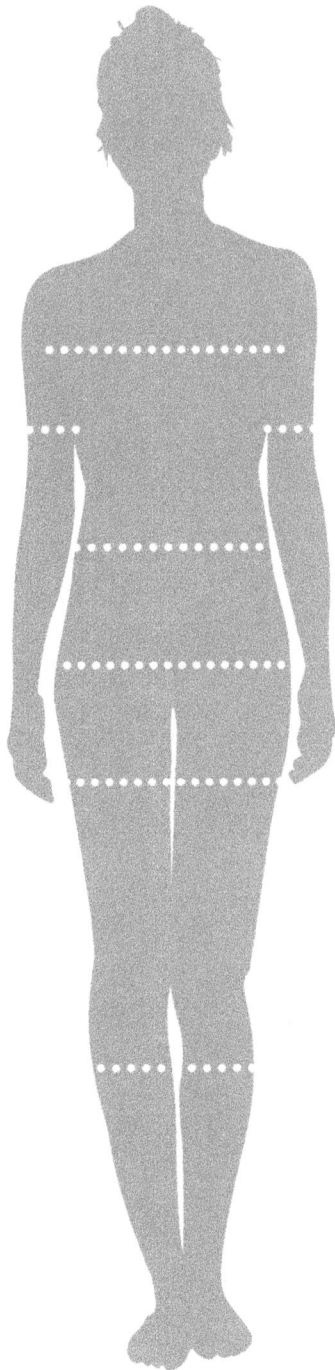

BEFORE	AFTER
DATE	DATE
CHEST	CHEST
LEFT ARM	LEFT ARM
RIGHT ARM	RIGHT ARM
WAIST	WAIST
HIPS	HIPS
LEFT THIGH	LEFT THIGH
RIGHT THIGH	
LEFT CALF	LEFT CALF
RIGHT CALF	RIGHT CALF
WEIGHT	WEIGHT

NOTES

BODY MEASUREMENTS TRACKER

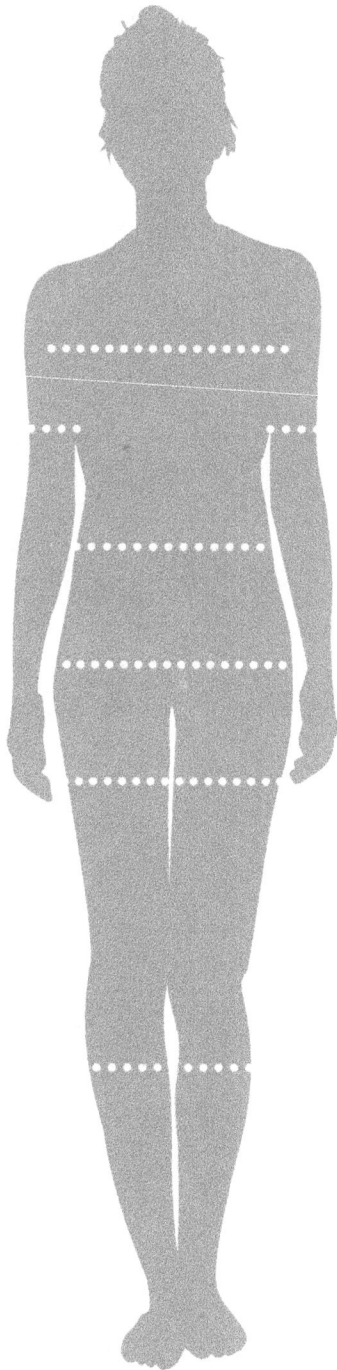

	BEFORE	AFTER
DATE		
CHEST		
LEFT ARM		
RIGHT ARM		
WAIST		
HIPS		
LEFT THIGH		
RIGHT THIGH		
LEFT CALF		
RIGHT CALF		
WEIGHT		
NOTES		

BODY MEASUREMENTS TRACKER

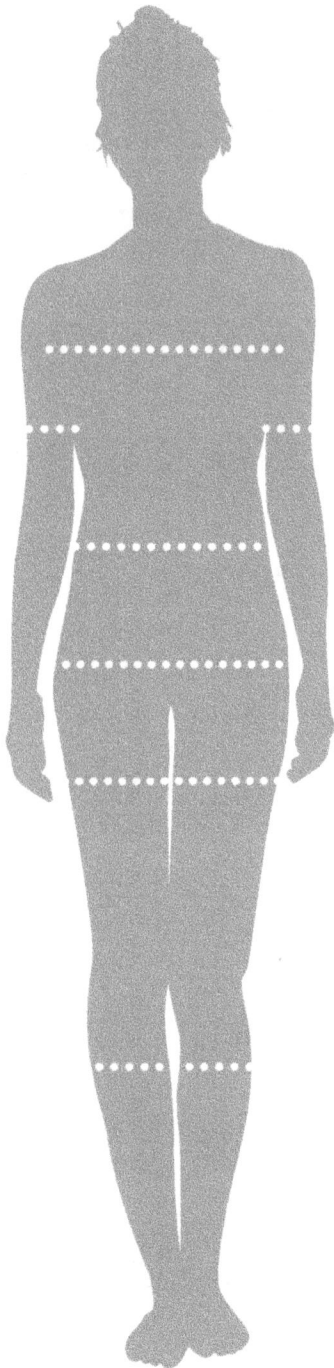

BEFORE

DATE

CHEST

LEFT ARM

RIGHT ARM

WAIST

HIPS

LEFT THIGH

RIGHT THIGH

LEFT CALF

RIGHT CALF

WEIGHT

NOTES

AFTER

DATE

CHEST

LEFT ARM

RIGHT ARM

WAIST

HIPS

LEFT THIGH

LEFT CALF

RIGHT CALF

WEIGHT

BODY MEASUREMENTS TRACKER

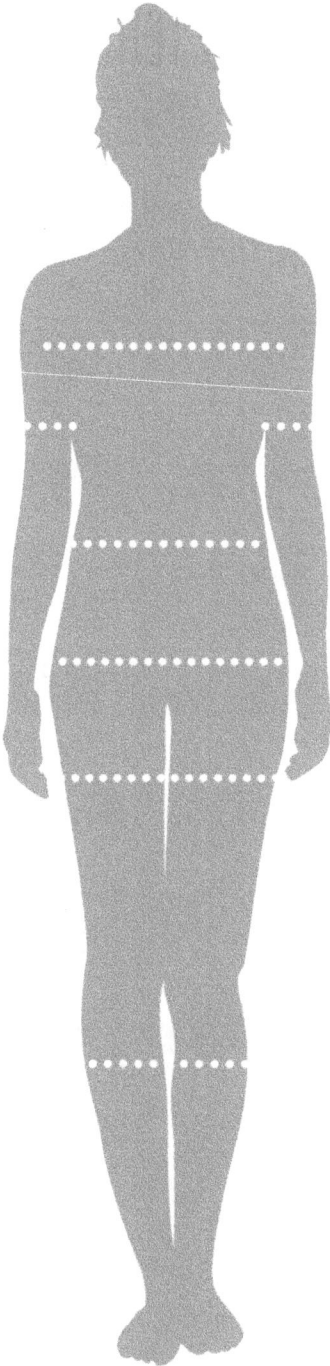

BEFORE

- DATE
- CHEST
- LEFT ARM
- RIGHT ARM
- WAIST
- HIPS
- LEFT THIGH
- RIGHT THIGH
- LEFT CALF
- RIGHT CALF
- WEIGHT
- NOTES

AFTER

- DATE
- CHEST
- LEFT ARM
- RIGHT ARM
- WAIST
- HIPS
- LEFT THIGH
- LEFT CALF
- RIGHT CALF
- WEIGHT

BODY MEASUREMENTS TRACKER

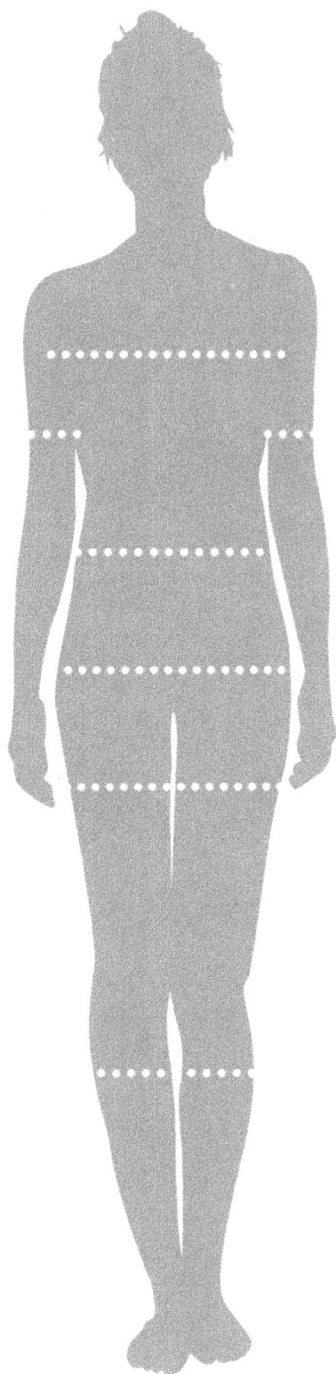

BEFORE

DATE

CHEST

LEFT ARM

RIGHT ARM

WAIST

HIPS

LEFT THIGH

RIGHT THIGH

LEFT CALF

RIGHT CALF

WEIGHT

NOTES

AFTER

DATE

CHEST

LEFT ARM

RIGHT ARM

WAIST

HIPS

LEFT THIGH

LEFT CALF

RIGHT CALF

WEIGHT

BODY MEASUREMENTS TRACKER

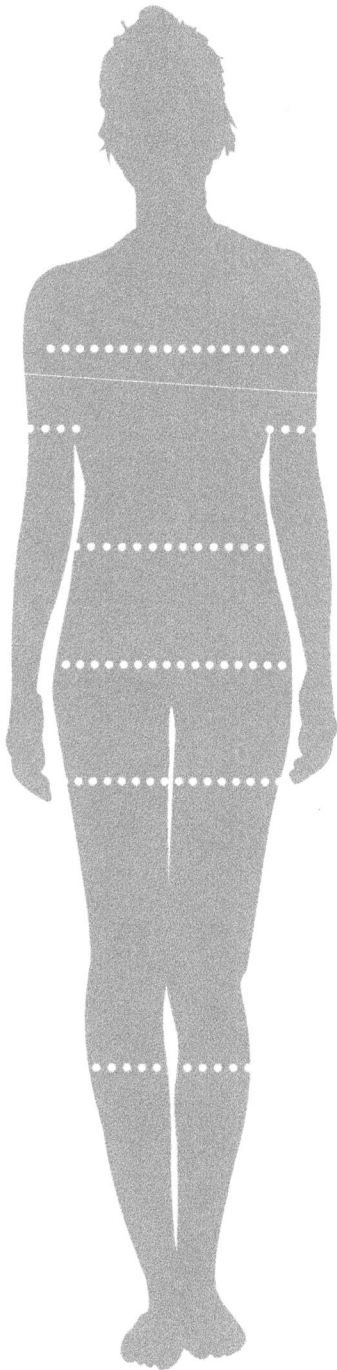

BEFORE

DATE

CHEST

LEFT ARM

RIGHT ARM

WAIST

HIPS

LEFT THIGH

RIGHT THIGH

LEFT CALF

RIGHT CALF

WEIGHT

NOTES

AFTER

DATE

CHEST

LEFT ARM

RIGHT ARM

WAIST

HIPS

LEFT THIGH

LEFT CALF

RIGHT CALF

WEIGHT

BODY MEASUREMENTS TRACKER

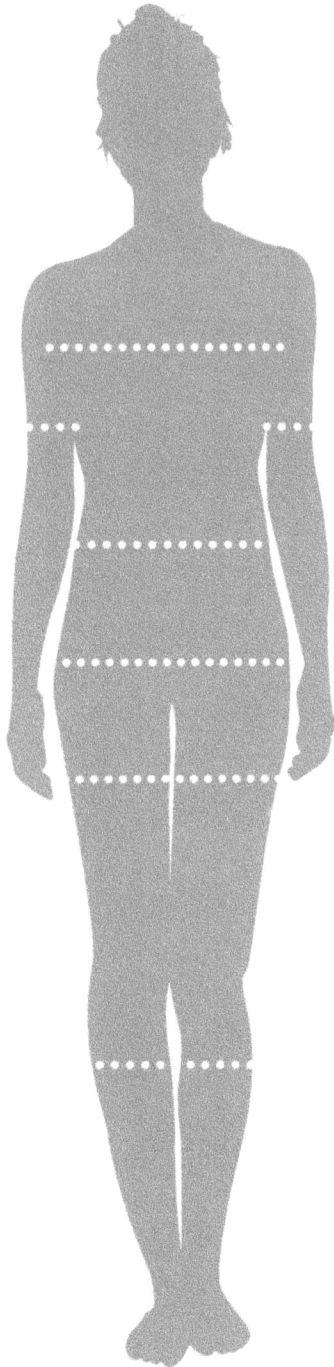

	BEFORE	AFTER
DATE		
CHEST		
LEFT ARM		
RIGHT ARM		
WAIST		
HIPS		
LEFT THIGH		
RIGHT THIGH		
LEFT CALF		
RIGHT CALF		
WEIGHT		
NOTES		

BODY MEASUREMENTS TRACKER

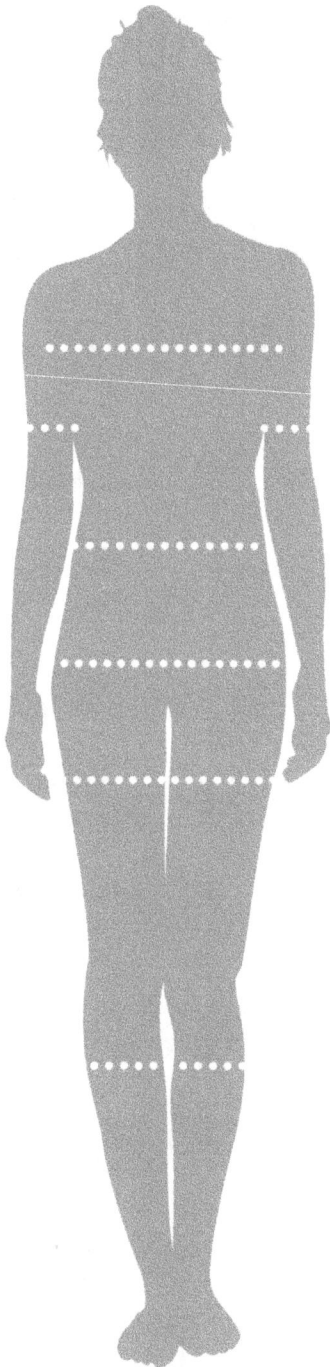

BEFORE

DATE

CHEST

LEFT ARM

RIGHT ARM

WAIST

HIPS

LEFT THIGH

RIGHT THIGH

LEFT CALF

RIGHT CALF

WEIGHT

NOTES

AFTER

DATE

CHEST

LEFT ARM

RIGHT ARM

WAIST

HIPS

LEFT THIGH

LEFT CALF

RIGHT CALF

WEIGHT

BODY MEASUREMENTS TRACKER

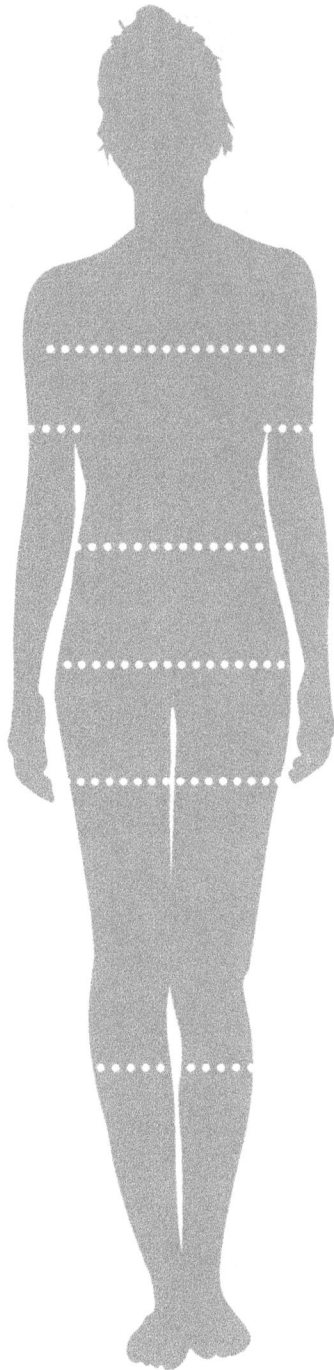

BEFORE

DATE

CHEST

LEFT ARM

RIGHT ARM

WAIST

HIPS

LEFT THIGH

RIGHT THIGH

LEFT CALF

RIGHT CALF

WEIGHT

NOTES

AFTER

DATE

CHEST

LEFT ARM

RIGHT ARM

WAIST

HIPS

LEFT THIGH

LEFT CALF

RIGHT CALF

WEIGHT

BODY MEASUREMENTS TRACKER

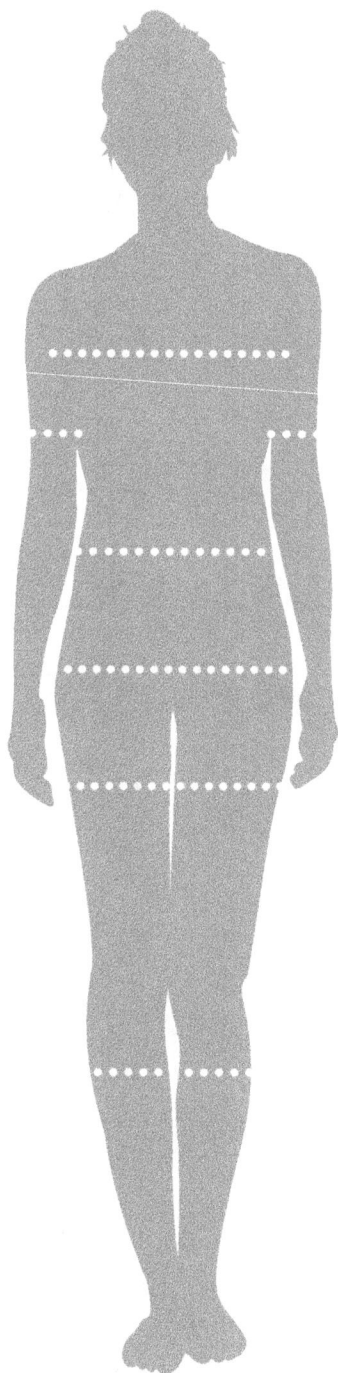

BEFORE

DATE

CHEST

LEFT ARM

RIGHT ARM

WAIST

HIPS

LEFT THIGH

RIGHT THIGH

LEFT CALF

RIGHT CALF

WEIGHT

NOTES

AFTER

DATE

CHEST

LEFT ARM

RIGHT ARM

WAIST

HIPS

LEFT THIGH

LEFT CALF

RIGHT CALF

WEIGHT

BODY MEASUREMENTS TRACKER

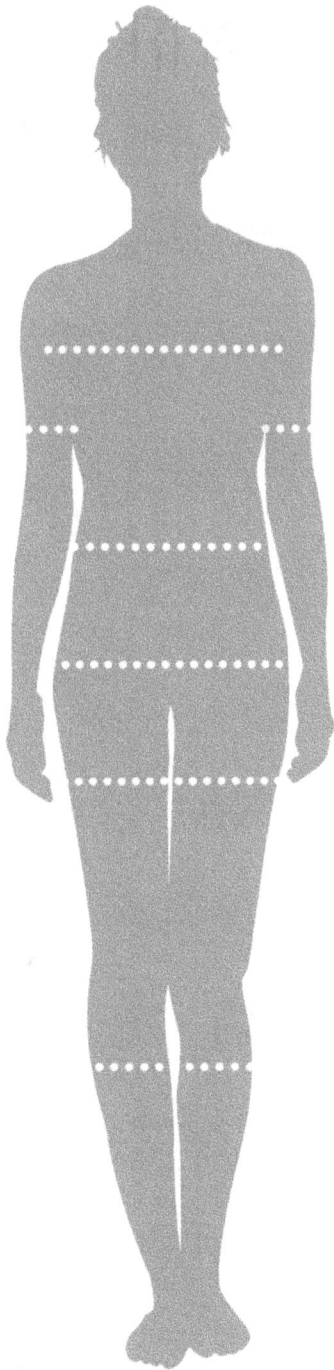

BEFORE

DATE

CHEST

LEFT ARM

RIGHT ARM

WAIST

HIPS

LEFT THIGH

RIGHT THIGH

LEFT CALF

RIGHT CALF

WEIGHT

NOTES

AFTER

DATE

CHEST

LEFT ARM

RIGHT ARM

WAIST

HIPS

LEFT THIGH

LEFT CALF

RIGHT CALF

WEIGHT

BODY MEASUREMENTS TRACKER

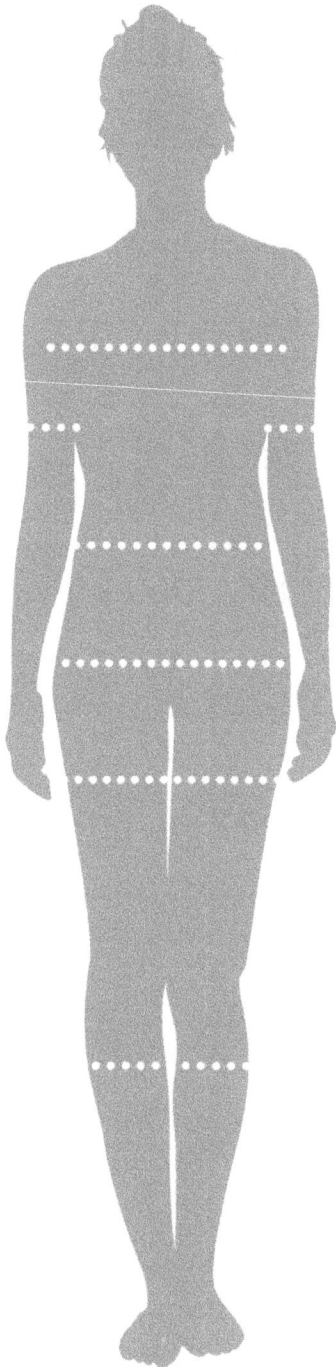

BEFORE

DATE

CHEST

LEFT ARM

RIGHT ARM

WAIST

HIPS

LEFT THIGH

RIGHT THIGH

LEFT CALF

RIGHT CALF

WEIGHT

NOTES

AFTER

DATE

CHEST

LEFT ARM

RIGHT ARM

WAIST

HIPS

LEFT THIGH

LEFT CALF

RIGHT CALF

WEIGHT

BODY MEASUREMENTS TRACKER

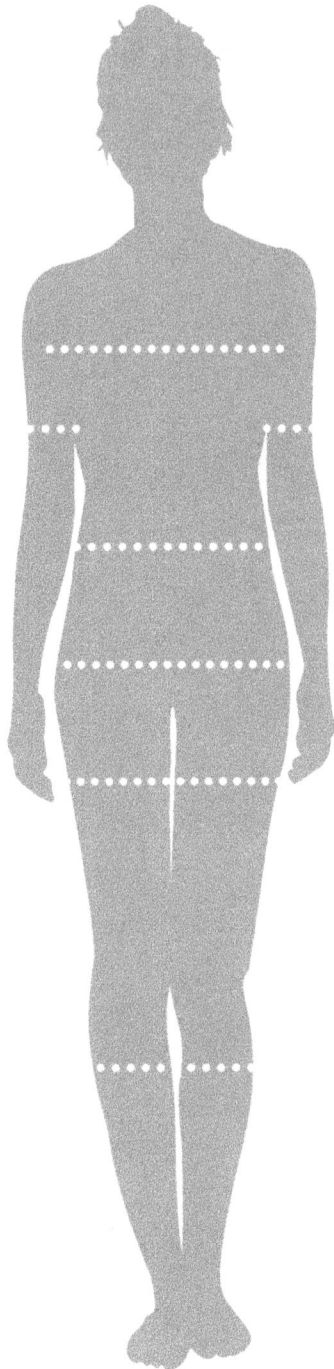

BEFORE

DATE	
CHEST	
LEFT ARM	
RIGHT ARM	
WAIST	
HIPS	
LEFT THIGH	
RIGHT THIGH	
LEFT CALF	
RIGHT CALF	
WEIGHT	

NOTES

AFTER

DATE	
CHEST	
LEFT ARM	
RIGHT ARM	
WAIST	
HIPS	
LEFT THIGH	
LEFT CALF	
RIGHT CALF	
WEIGHT	

BODY MEASUREMENTS TRACKER

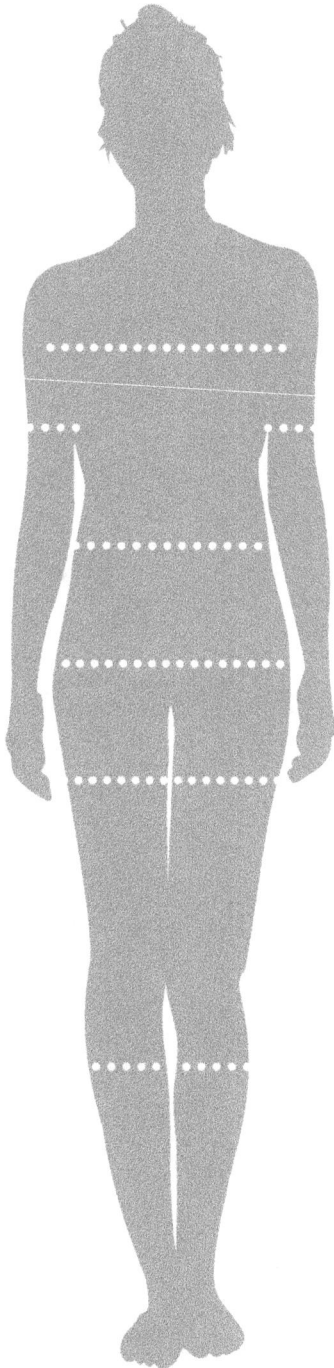

BEFORE

DATE

CHEST

LEFT ARM

RIGHT ARM

WAIST

HIPS

LEFT THIGH

RIGHT THIGH

LEFT CALF

RIGHT CALF

WEIGHT

NOTES

AFTER

DATE

CHEST

LEFT ARM

RIGHT ARM

WAIST

HIPS

LEFT THIGH

LEFT CALF

RIGHT CALF

WEIGHT

BODY MEASUREMENTS TRACKER

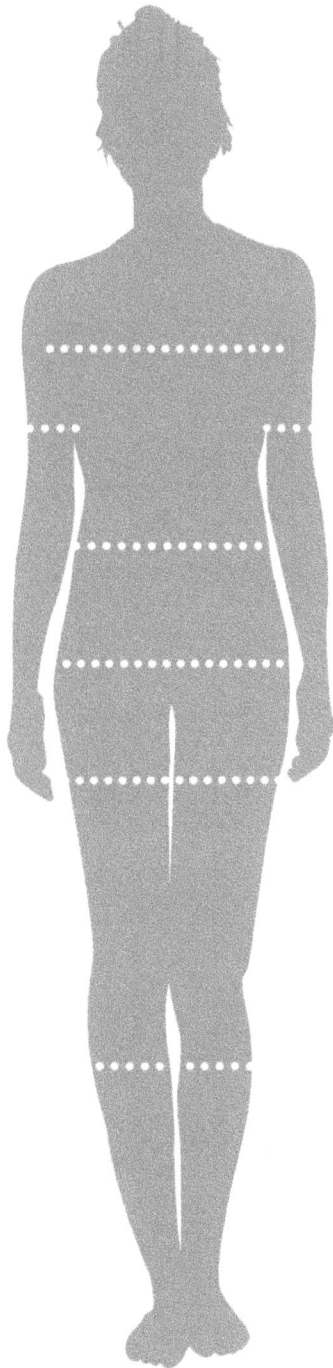

BEFORE

DATE	
CHEST	
LEFT ARM	
RIGHT ARM	
WAIST	
HIPS	
LEFT THIGH	
RIGHT THIGH	
LEFT CALF	
RIGHT CALF	
WEIGHT	

AFTER

DATE	
CHEST	
LEFT ARM	
RIGHT ARM	
WAIST	
HIPS	
LEFT THIGH	
LEFT CALF	
RIGHT CALF	
WEIGHT	

NOTES

BODY MEASUREMENTS TRACKER

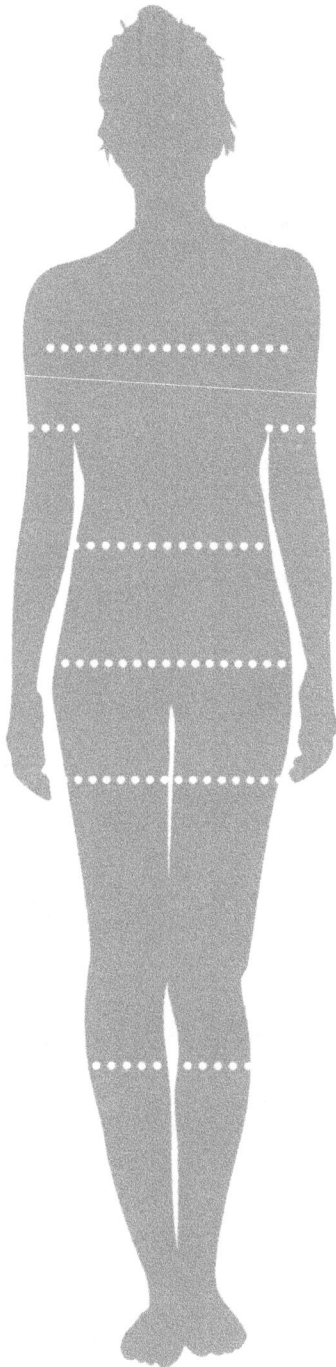

BEFORE

DATE

CHEST

LEFT ARM

RIGHT ARM

WAIST

HIPS

LEFT THIGH

RIGHT THIGH

LEFT CALF

RIGHT CALF

WEIGHT

NOTES

AFTER

DATE

CHEST

LEFT ARM

RIGHT ARM

WAIST

HIPS

LEFT THIGH

LEFT CALF

RIGHT CALF

WEIGHT

BODY MEASUREMENTS TRACKER

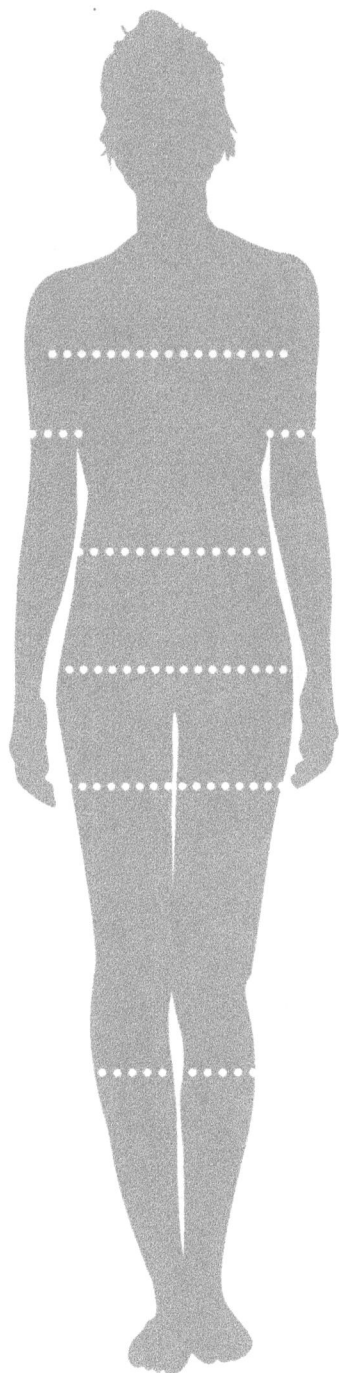

BEFORE

DATE

CHEST

LEFT ARM

RIGHT ARM

WAIST

HIPS

LEFT THIGH

RIGHT THIGH

LEFT CALF

RIGHT CALF

WEIGHT

NOTES

AFTER

DATE

CHEST

LEFT ARM

RIGHT ARM

WAIST

HIPS

LEFT THIGH

LEFT CALF

RIGHT CALF

WEIGHT

BODY MEASUREMENTS TRACKER

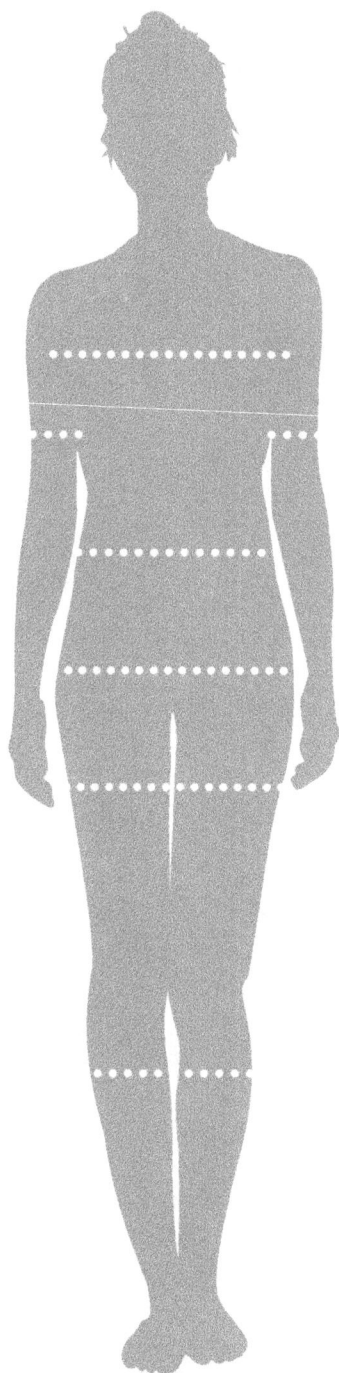

BEFORE

- DATE
- CHEST
- LEFT ARM
- RIGHT ARM
- WAIST
- HIPS
- LEFT THIGH
- RIGHT THIGH
- LEFT CALF
- RIGHT CALF
- WEIGHT
- NOTES

AFTER

- DATE
- CHEST
- LEFT ARM
- RIGHT ARM
- WAIST
- HIPS
- LEFT THIGH
- LEFT CALF
- RIGHT CALF
- WEIGHT

BODY MEASUREMENTS TRACKER

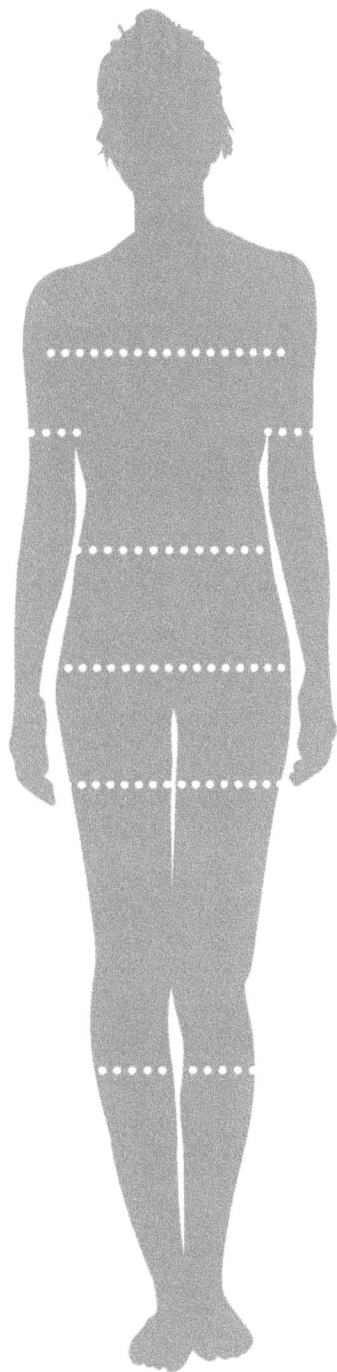

BEFORE	AFTER
DATE	DATE
CHEST	CHEST
LEFT ARM	LEFT ARM
RIGHT ARM	RIGHT ARM
WAIST	WAIST
HIPS	HIPS
LEFT THIGH	LEFT THIGH
RIGHT THIGH	
LEFT CALF	LEFT CALF
RIGHT CALF	RIGHT CALF
WEIGHT	WEIGHT
NOTES	

BODY MEASUREMENTS TRACKER

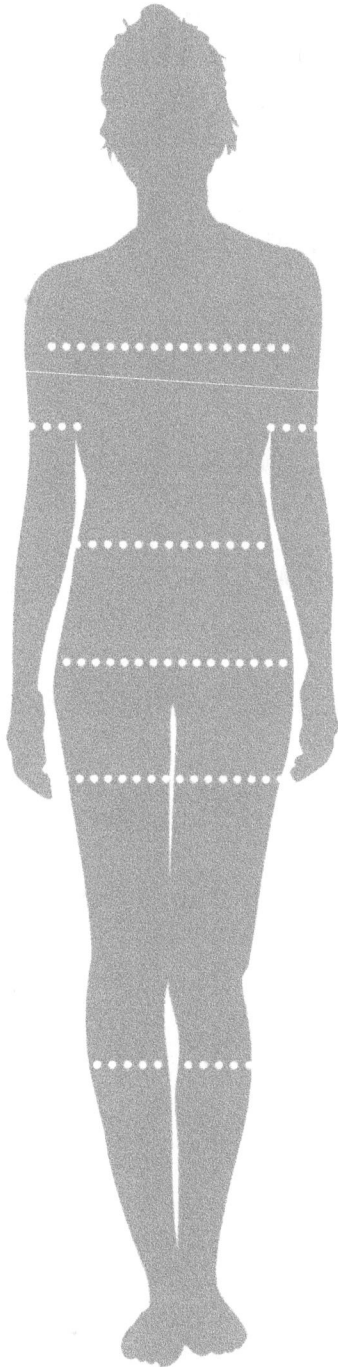

BEFORE

DATE

CHEST

LEFT ARM

RIGHT ARM

WAIST

HIPS

LEFT THIGH

RIGHT THIGH

LEFT CALF

RIGHT CALF

WEIGHT

NOTES

AFTER

DATE

CHEST

LEFT ARM

RIGHT ARM

WAIST

HIPS

LEFT THIGH

LEFT CALF

RIGHT CALF

WEIGHT

BODY MEASUREMENTS TRACKER

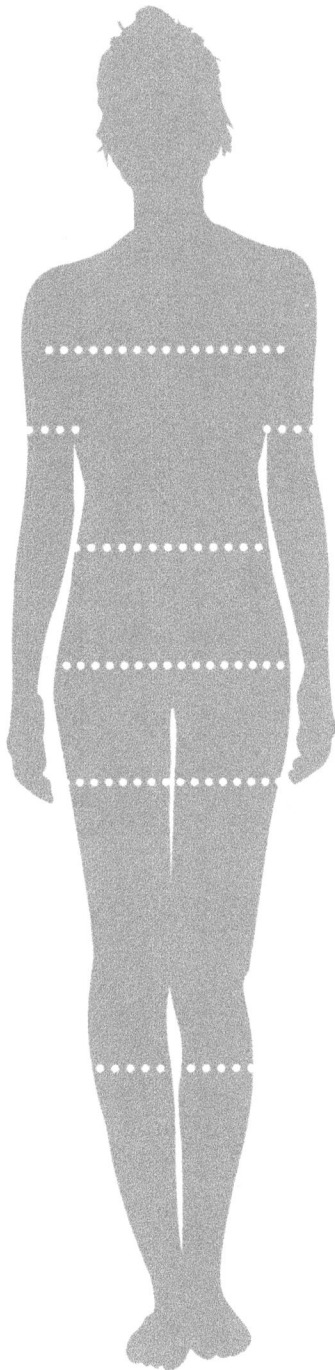

BEFORE

DATE	
CHEST	
LEFT ARM	
RIGHT ARM	
WAIST	
HIPS	
LEFT THIGH	
RIGHT THIGH	
LEFT CALF	
RIGHT CALF	
WEIGHT	

AFTER

DATE	
CHEST	
LEFT ARM	
RIGHT ARM	
WAIST	
HIPS	
LEFT THIGH	
LEFT CALF	
RIGHT CALF	
WEIGHT	

NOTES

BODY MEASUREMENTS TRACKER

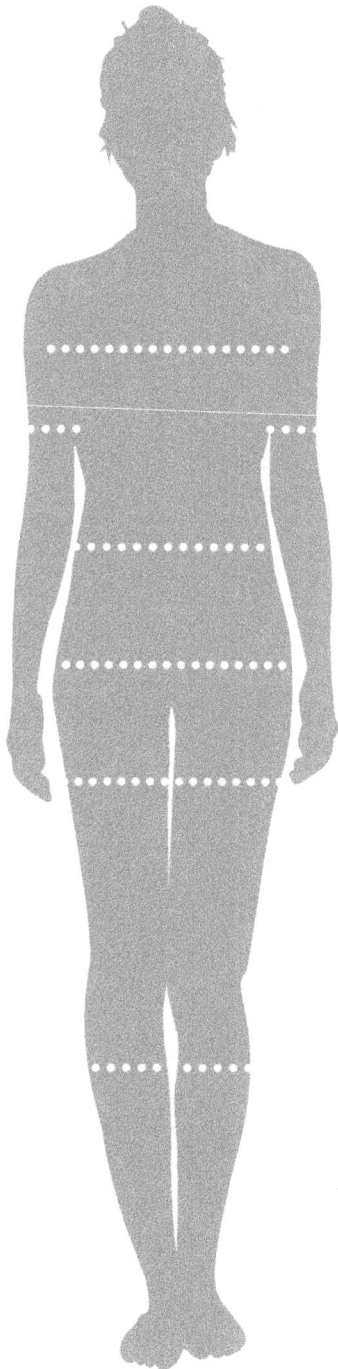

BEFORE

DATE

CHEST

LEFT ARM

RIGHT ARM

WAIST

HIPS

LEFT THIGH

RIGHT THIGH

LEFT CALF

RIGHT CALF

WEIGHT

NOTES

AFTER

DATE

CHEST

LEFT ARM

RIGHT ARM

WAIST

HIPS

LEFT THIGH

LEFT CALF

RIGHT CALF

WEIGHT

BODY MEASUREMENTS TRACKER

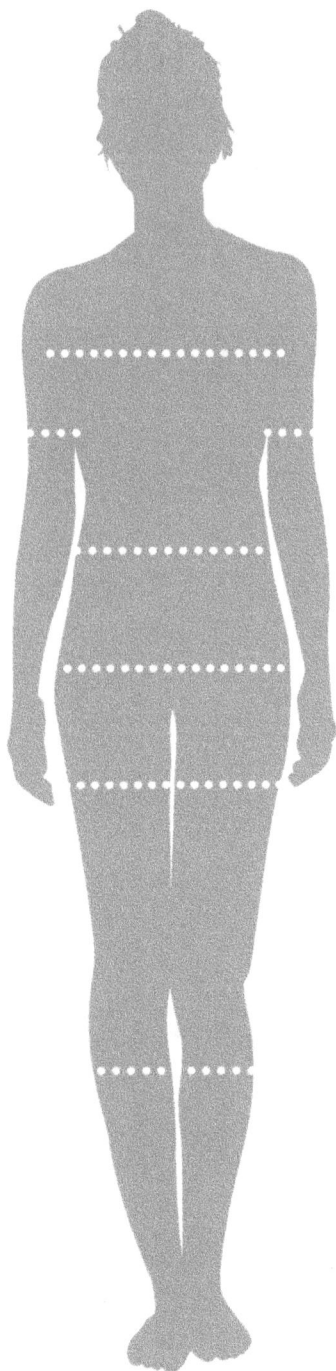

BEFORE

DATE

CHEST

LEFT ARM

RIGHT ARM

WAIST

HIPS

LEFT THIGH

RIGHT THIGH

LEFT CALF

RIGHT CALF

WEIGHT

NOTES

AFTER

DATE

CHEST

LEFT ARM

RIGHT ARM

WAIST

HIPS

LEFT THIGH

LEFT CALF

RIGHT CALF

WEIGHT

BODY MEASUREMENTS TRACKER

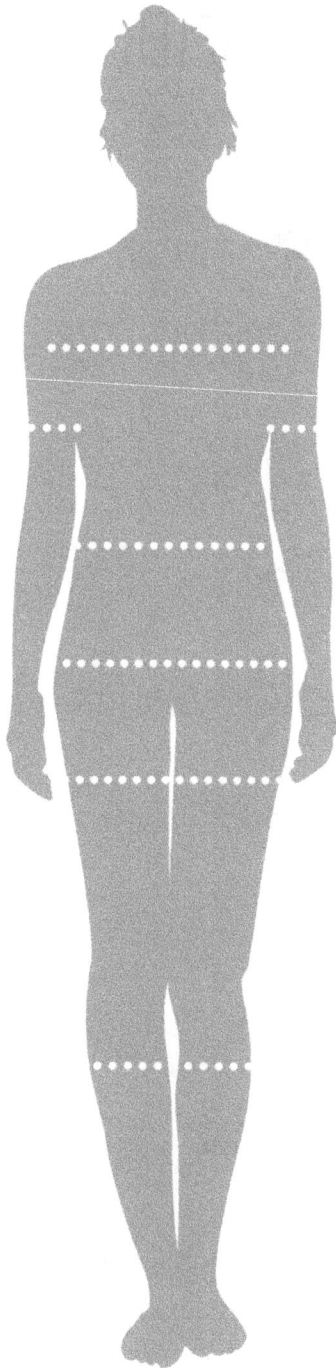

BEFORE

DATE

CHEST

LEFT ARM

RIGHT ARM

WAIST

HIPS

LEFT THIGH

RIGHT THIGH

LEFT CALF

RIGHT CALF

WEIGHT

NOTES

AFTER

DATE

CHEST

LEFT ARM

RIGHT ARM

WAIST

HIPS

LEFT THIGH

LEFT CALF

RIGHT CALF

WEIGHT

BODY MEASUREMENTS TRACKER

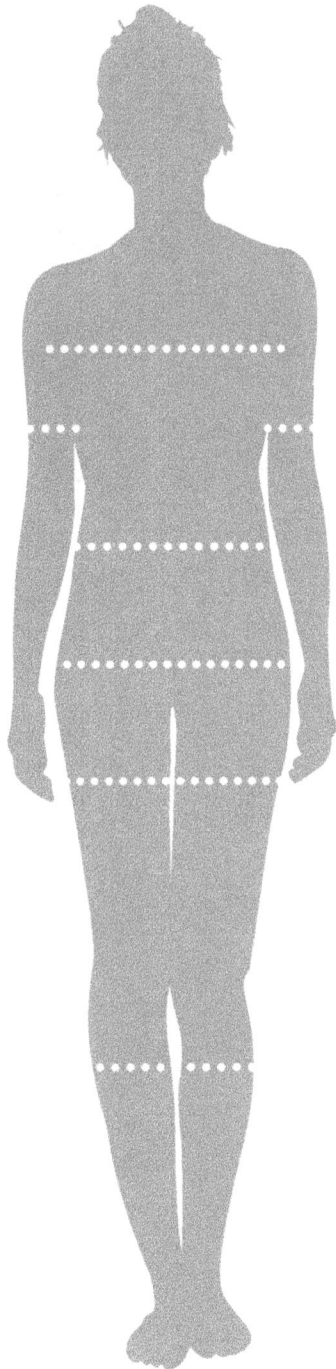

BEFORE

DATE

CHEST

LEFT ARM

RIGHT ARM

WAIST

HIPS

LEFT THIGH

RIGHT THIGH

LEFT CALF

RIGHT CALF

WEIGHT

NOTES

AFTER

DATE

CHEST

LEFT ARM

RIGHT ARM

WAIST

HIPS

LEFT THIGH

LEFT CALF

RIGHT CALF

WEIGHT

BODY MEASUREMENTS TRACKER

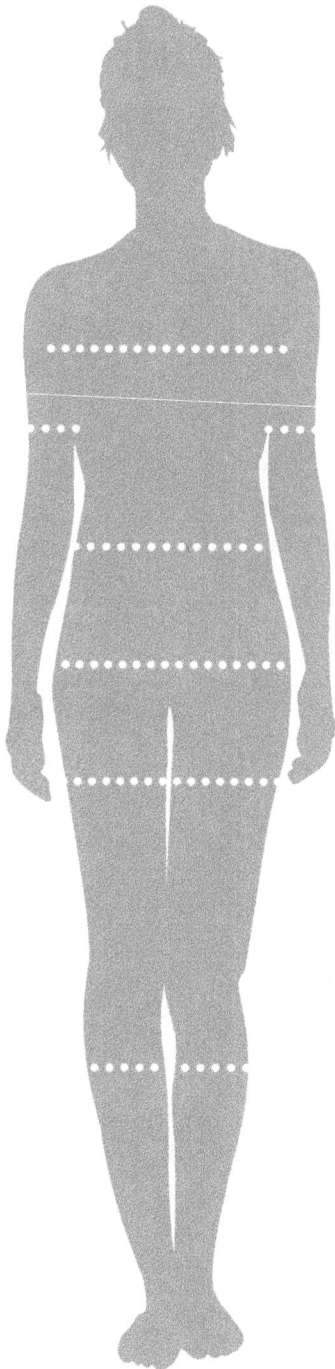

BEFORE

DATE

CHEST

LEFT ARM

RIGHT ARM

WAIST

HIPS

LEFT THIGH

RIGHT THIGH

LEFT CALF

RIGHT CALF

WEIGHT

NOTES

AFTER

DATE

CHEST

LEFT ARM

RIGHT ARM

WAIST

HIPS

LEFT THIGH

LEFT CALF

RIGHT CALF

WEIGHT

BODY MEASUREMENTS TRACKER

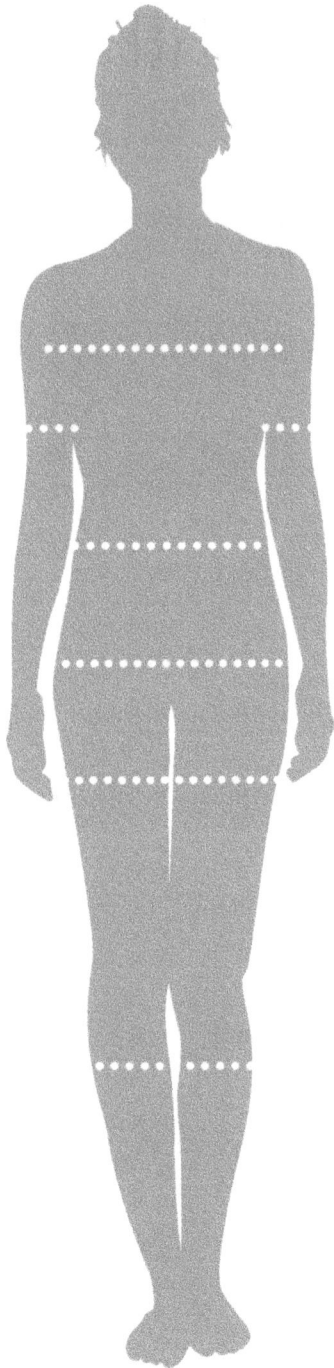

BEFORE

DATE	
CHEST	
LEFT ARM	
RIGHT ARM	
WAIST	
HIPS	
LEFT THIGH	
RIGHT THIGH	
LEFT CALF	
RIGHT CALF	
WEIGHT	

AFTER

DATE	
CHEST	
LEFT ARM	
RIGHT ARM	
WAIST	
HIPS	
LEFT THIGH	
LEFT CALF	
RIGHT CALF	
WEIGHT	

NOTES

BODY MEASUREMENTS TRACKER

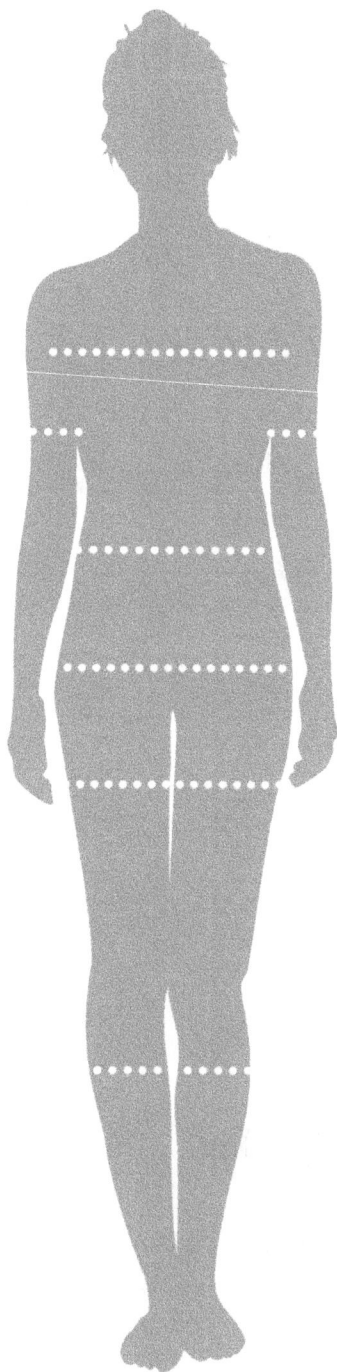

BEFORE

DATE

CHEST

LEFT ARM

RIGHT ARM

WAIST

HIPS

LEFT THIGH

RIGHT THIGH

LEFT CALF

RIGHT CALF

WEIGHT

NOTES

AFTER

DATE

CHEST

LEFT ARM

RIGHT ARM

WAIST

HIPS

LEFT THIGH

LEFT CALF

RIGHT CALF

WEIGHT

BODY MEASUREMENTS TRACKER

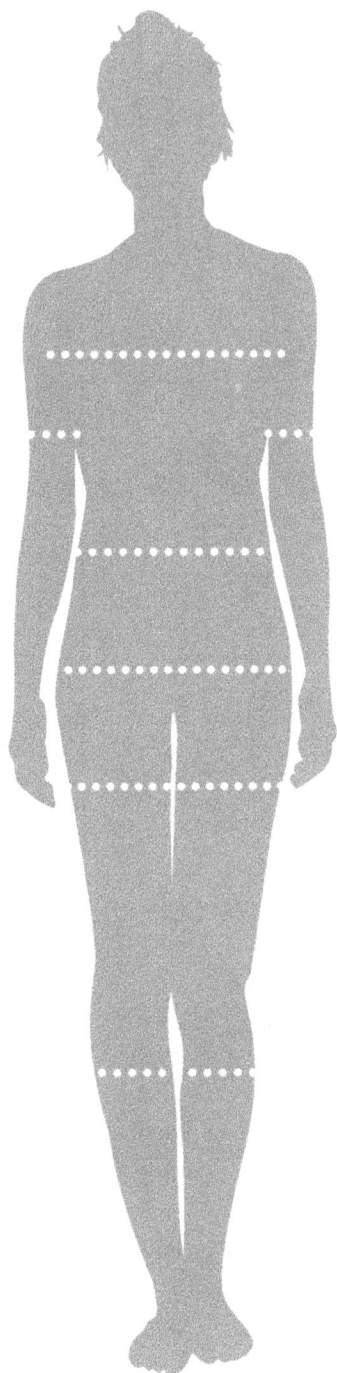

BEFORE

- DATE
- CHEST
- LEFT ARM
- RIGHT ARM
- WAIST
- HIPS
- LEFT THIGH
- RIGHT THIGH
- LEFT CALF
- RIGHT CALF
- WEIGHT
- NOTES

AFTER

- DATE
- CHEST
- LEFT ARM
- RIGHT ARM
- WAIST
- HIPS
- LEFT THIGH
- LEFT CALF
- RIGHT CALF
- WEIGHT

BODY MEASUREMENTS TRACKER

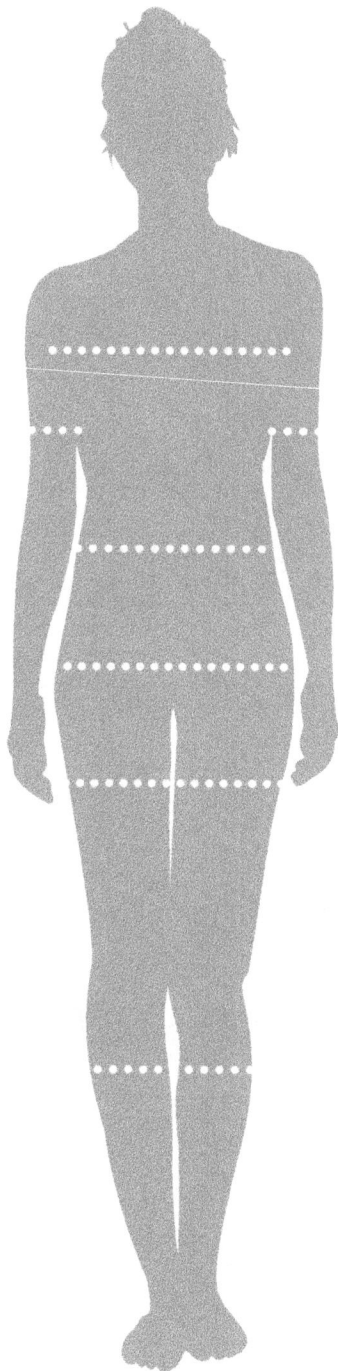

BEFORE

DATE

CHEST

LEFT ARM

RIGHT ARM

WAIST

HIPS

LEFT THIGH

RIGHT THIGH

LEFT CALF

RIGHT CALF

WEIGHT

NOTES

AFTER

DATE

CHEST

LEFT ARM

RIGHT ARM

WAIST

HIPS

LEFT THIGH

LEFT CALF

RIGHT CALF

WEIGHT

BODY MEASUREMENTS TRACKER

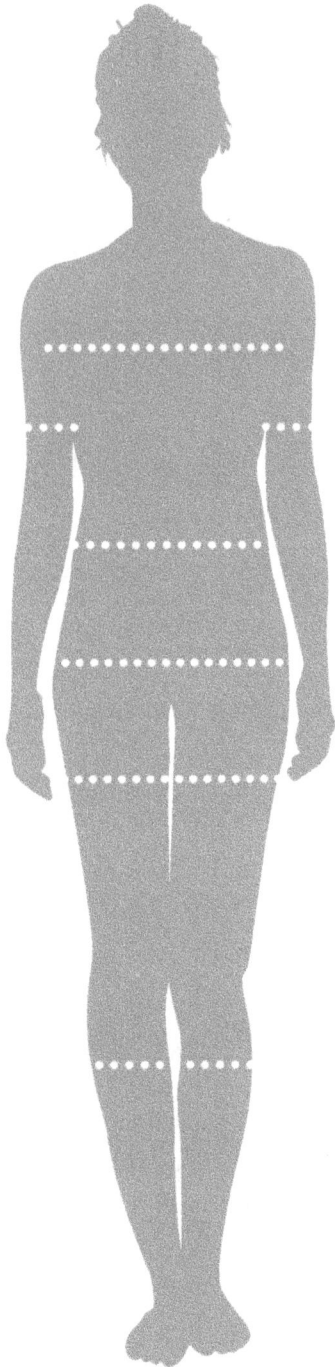

	BEFORE	AFTER
DATE		
CHEST		
LEFT ARM		
RIGHT ARM		
WAIST		
HIPS		
LEFT THIGH		
RIGHT THIGH		
LEFT CALF		
RIGHT CALF		
WEIGHT		
NOTES		

BODY MEASUREMENTS TRACKER

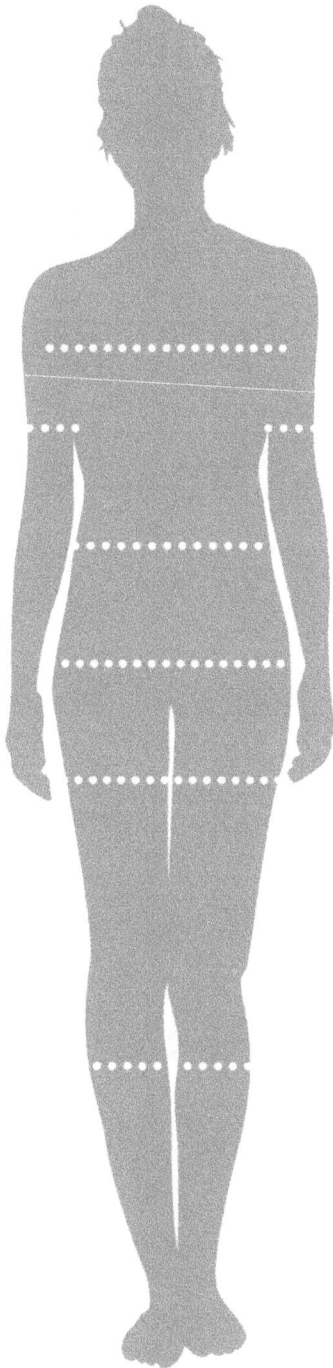

BEFORE

DATE

CHEST

LEFT ARM

RIGHT ARM

WAIST

HIPS

LEFT THIGH

RIGHT THIGH

LEFT CALF

RIGHT CALF

WEIGHT

NOTES

AFTER

DATE

CHEST

LEFT ARM

RIGHT ARM

WAIST

HIPS

LEFT THIGH

LEFT CALF

RIGHT CALF

WEIGHT

BODY MEASUREMENTS TRACKER

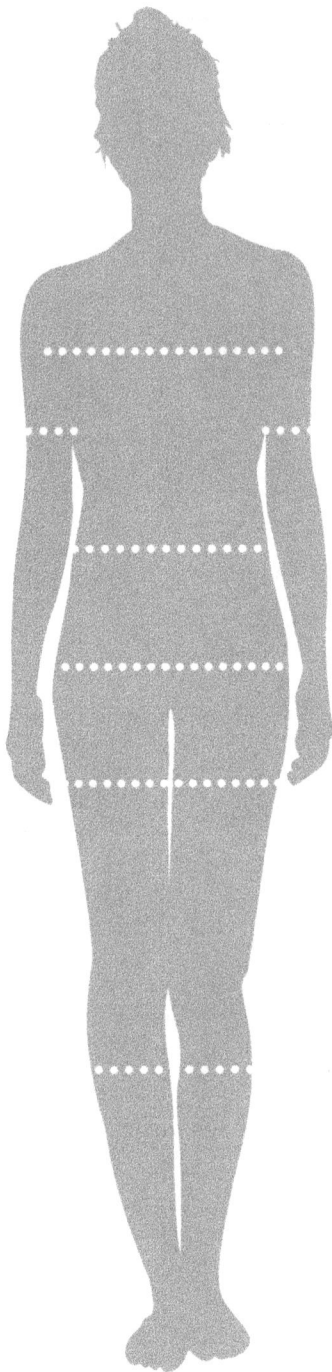

BEFORE

DATE

CHEST

LEFT ARM

RIGHT ARM

WAIST

HIPS

LEFT THIGH

RIGHT THIGH

LEFT CALF

RIGHT CALF

WEIGHT

NOTES

AFTER

DATE

CHEST

LEFT ARM

RIGHT ARM

WAIST

HIPS

LEFT THIGH

LEFT CALF

RIGHT CALF

WEIGHT

BODY MEASUREMENTS TRACKER

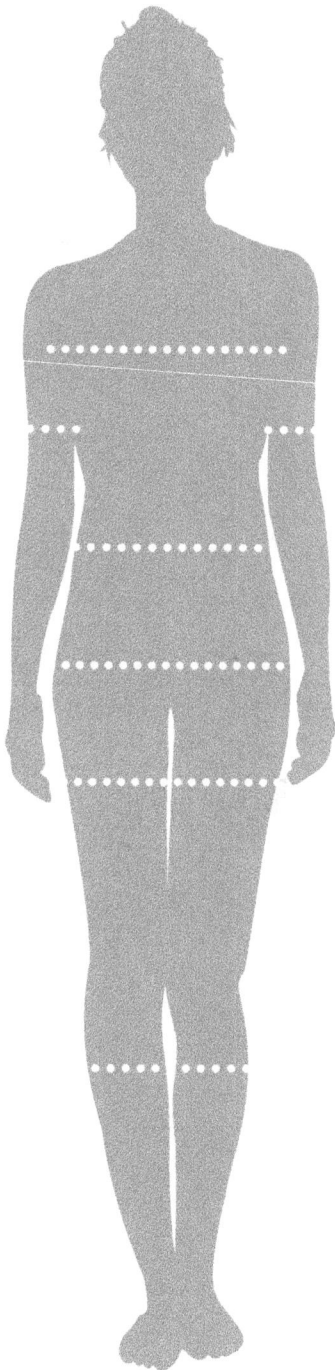

BEFORE

DATE

CHEST

LEFT ARM

RIGHT ARM

WAIST

HIPS

LEFT THIGH

RIGHT THIGH

LEFT CALF

RIGHT CALF

WEIGHT

NOTES

AFTER

DATE

CHEST

LEFT ARM

RIGHT ARM

WAIST

HIPS

LEFT THIGH

LEFT CALF

RIGHT CALF

WEIGHT

BODY MEASUREMENTS TRACKER

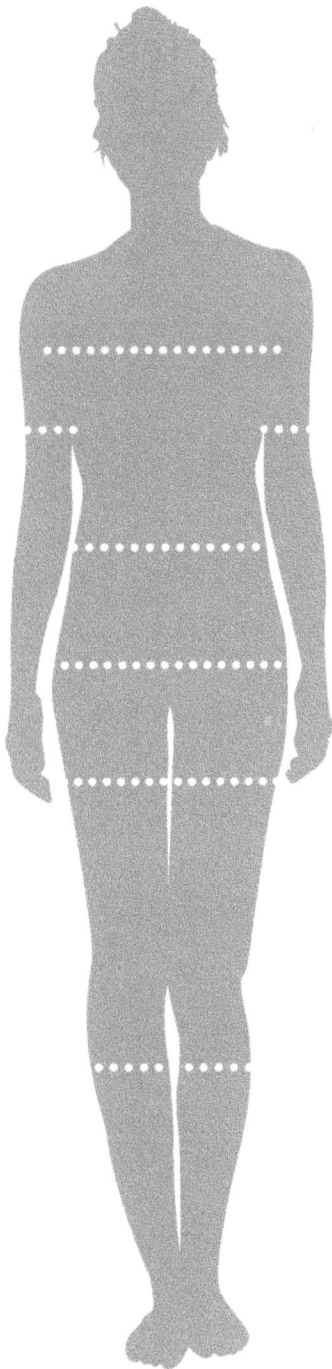

BEFORE

DATE

CHEST

LEFT ARM

RIGHT ARM

WAIST

HIPS

LEFT THIGH

RIGHT THIGH

LEFT CALF

RIGHT CALF

WEIGHT

NOTES

AFTER

DATE

CHEST

LEFT ARM

RIGHT ARM

WAIST

HIPS

LEFT THIGH

LEFT CALF

RIGHT CALF

WEIGHT

BODY MEASUREMENTS TRACKER

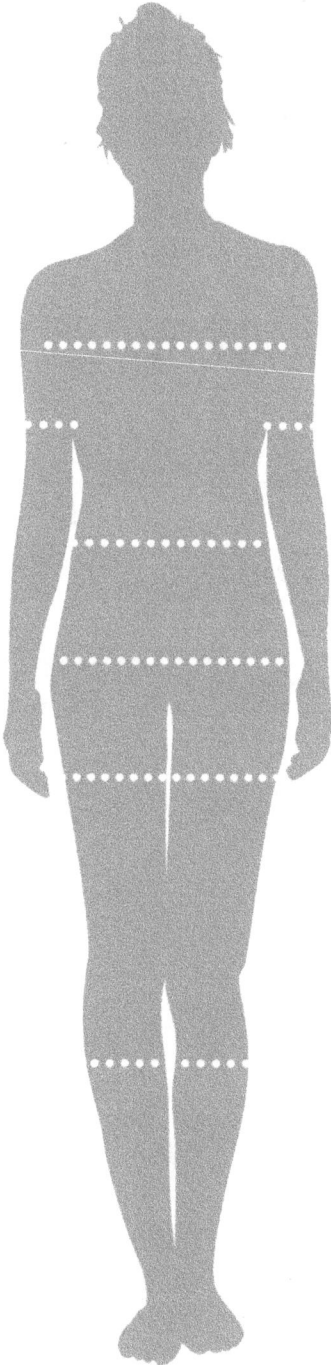

BEFORE

DATE

CHEST

LEFT ARM

RIGHT ARM

WAIST

HIPS

LEFT THIGH

RIGHT THIGH

LEFT CALF

RIGHT CALF

WEIGHT

NOTES

AFTER

DATE

CHEST

LEFT ARM

RIGHT ARM

WAIST

HIPS

LEFT THIGH

LEFT CALF

RIGHT CALF

WEIGHT

BODY MEASUREMENTS TRACKER

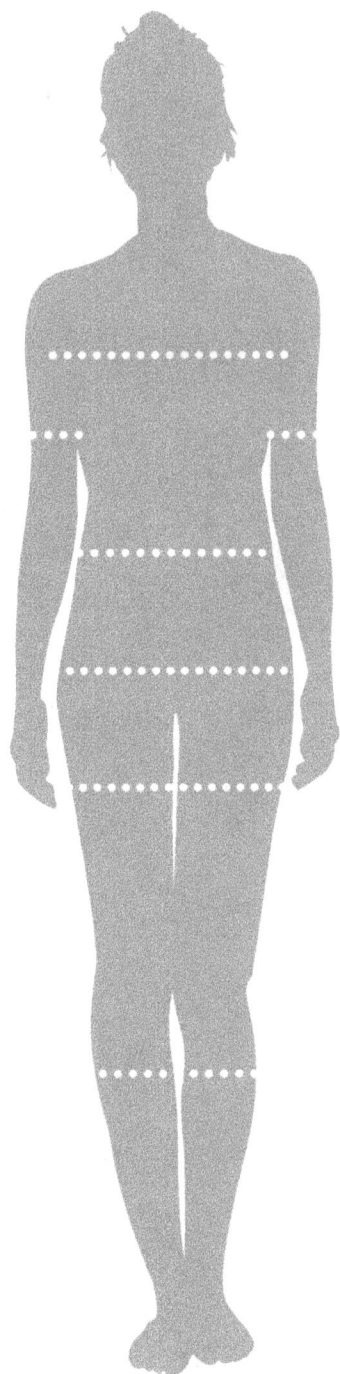

BEFORE

DATE

CHEST

LEFT ARM

RIGHT ARM

WAIST

HIPS

LEFT THIGH

RIGHT THIGH

LEFT CALF

RIGHT CALF

WEIGHT

NOTES

AFTER

DATE

CHEST

LEFT ARM

RIGHT ARM

WAIST

HIPS

LEFT THIGH

LEFT CALF

RIGHT CALF

WEIGHT

BODY MEASUREMENTS TRACKER

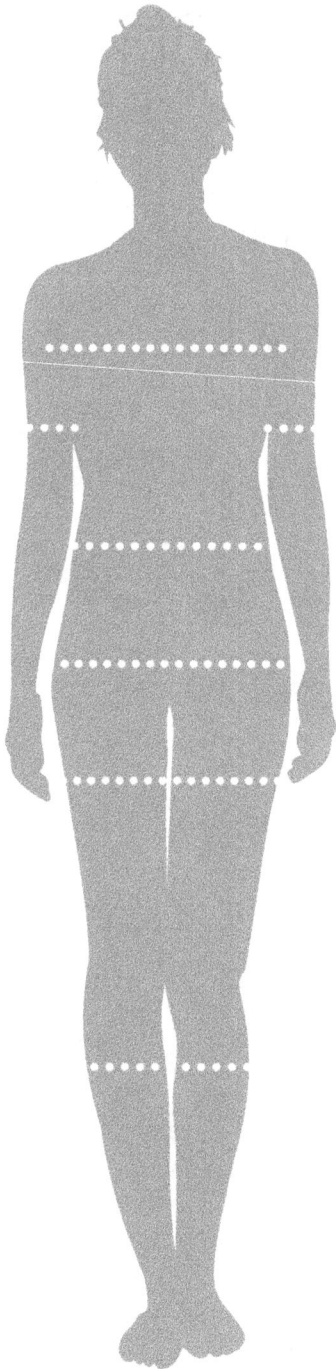

BEFORE

DATE

CHEST

LEFT ARM

RIGHT ARM

WAIST

HIPS

LEFT THIGH

RIGHT THIGH

LEFT CALF

RIGHT CALF

WEIGHT

NOTES

AFTER

DATE

CHEST

LEFT ARM

RIGHT ARM

WAIST

HIPS

LEFT THIGH

LEFT CALF

RIGHT CALF

WEIGHT

BODY MEASUREMENTS TRACKER

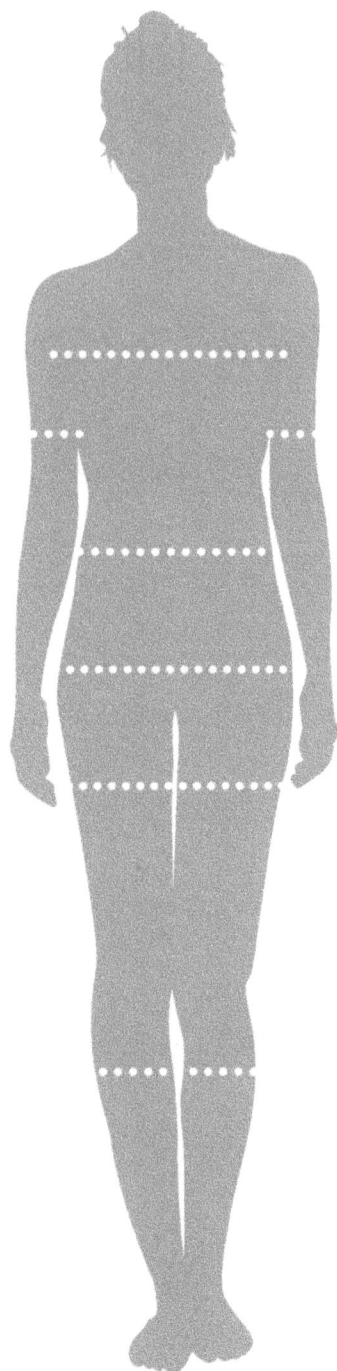

BEFORE

DATE

CHEST

LEFT ARM

RIGHT ARM

WAIST

HIPS

LEFT THIGH

RIGHT THIGH

LEFT CALF

RIGHT CALF

WEIGHT

NOTES

AFTER

DATE

CHEST

LEFT ARM

RIGHT ARM

WAIST

HIPS

LEFT THIGH

LEFT CALF

RIGHT CALF

WEIGHT

BODY MEASUREMENTS TRACKER

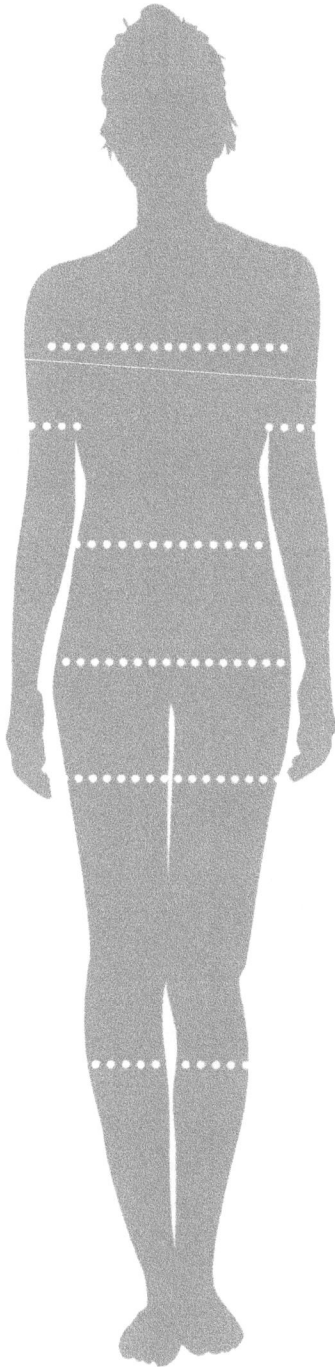

BEFORE

DATE

CHEST

LEFT ARM

RIGHT ARM

WAIST

HIPS

LEFT THIGH

RIGHT THIGH

LEFT CALF

RIGHT CALF

WEIGHT

NOTES

AFTER

DATE

CHEST

LEFT ARM

RIGHT ARM

WAIST

HIPS

LEFT THIGH

LEFT CALF

RIGHT CALF

WEIGHT

BODY MEASUREMENTS TRACKER

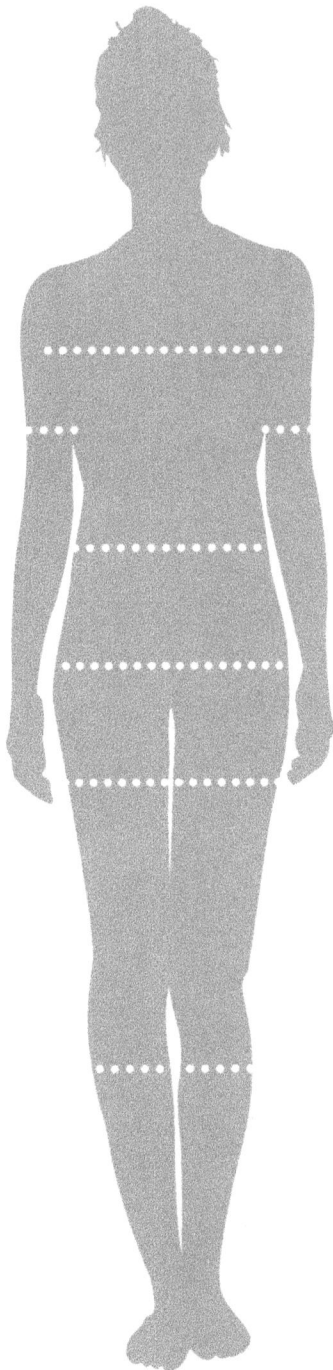

BEFORE

DATE

CHEST

LEFT ARM

RIGHT ARM

WAIST

HIPS

LEFT THIGH

RIGHT THIGH

LEFT CALF

RIGHT CALF

WEIGHT

NOTES

AFTER

DATE

CHEST

LEFT ARM

RIGHT ARM

WAIST

HIPS

LEFT THIGH

LEFT CALF

RIGHT CALF

WEIGHT

BODY MEASUREMENTS TRACKER

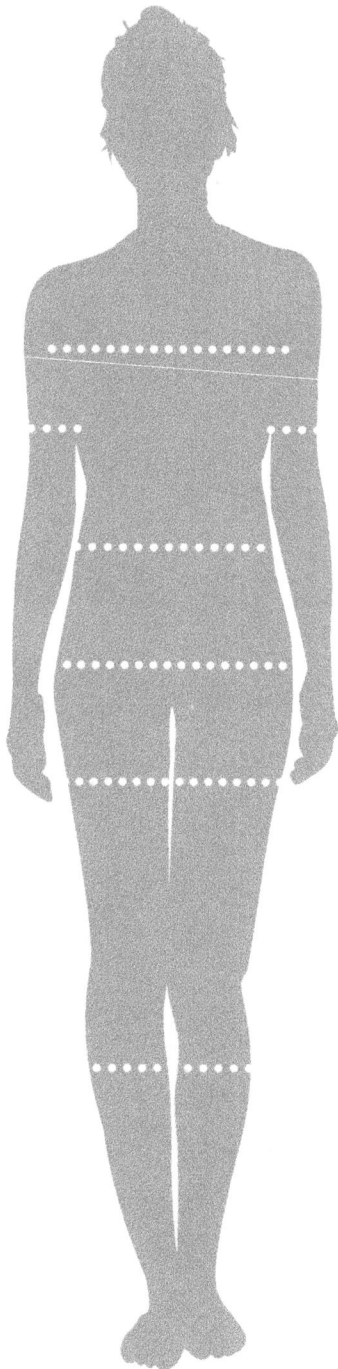

BEFORE

DATE

CHEST

LEFT ARM

RIGHT ARM

WAIST

HIPS

LEFT THIGH

RIGHT THIGH

LEFT CALF

RIGHT CALF

WEIGHT

NOTES

AFTER

DATE

CHEST

LEFT ARM

RIGHT ARM

WAIST

HIPS

LEFT THIGH

LEFT CALF

RIGHT CALF

WEIGHT

BODY MEASUREMENTS TRACKER

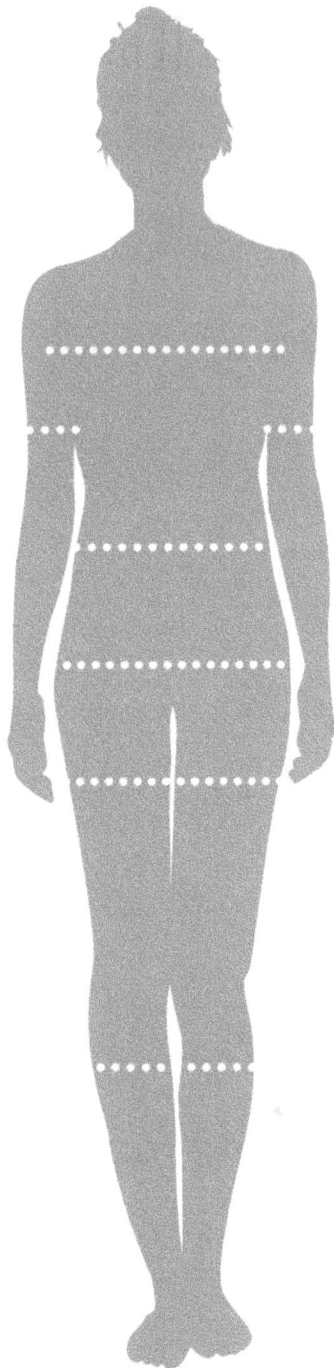

BEFORE

DATE

CHEST

LEFT ARM

RIGHT ARM

WAIST

HIPS

LEFT THIGH

RIGHT THIGH

LEFT CALF

RIGHT CALF

WEIGHT

NOTES

AFTER

DATE

CHEST

LEFT ARM

RIGHT ARM

WAIST

HIPS

LEFT THIGH

LEFT CALF

RIGHT CALF

WEIGHT

BODY MEASUREMENTS TRACKER

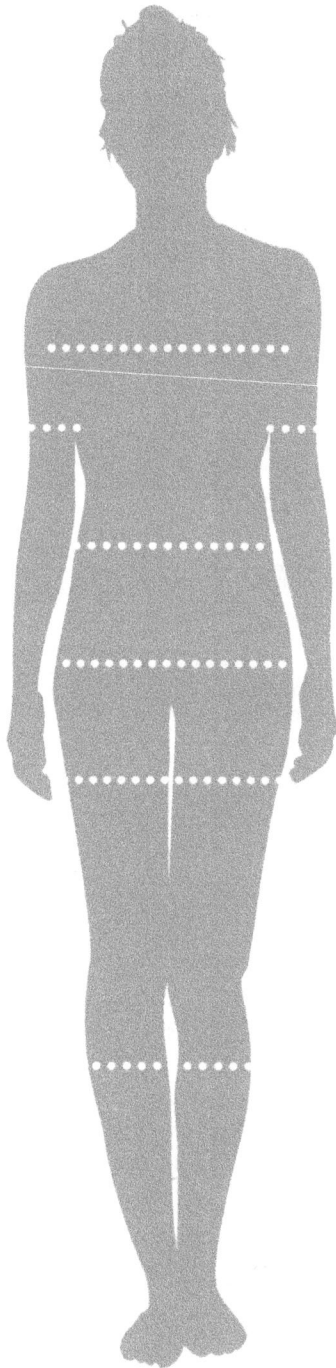

BEFORE

DATE

CHEST

LEFT ARM

RIGHT ARM

WAIST

HIPS

LEFT THIGH

RIGHT THIGH

LEFT CALF

RIGHT CALF

WEIGHT

NOTES

AFTER

DATE

CHEST

LEFT ARM

RIGHT ARM

WAIST

HIPS

LEFT THIGH

LEFT CALF

RIGHT CALF

WEIGHT

BODY MEASUREMENTS TRACKER

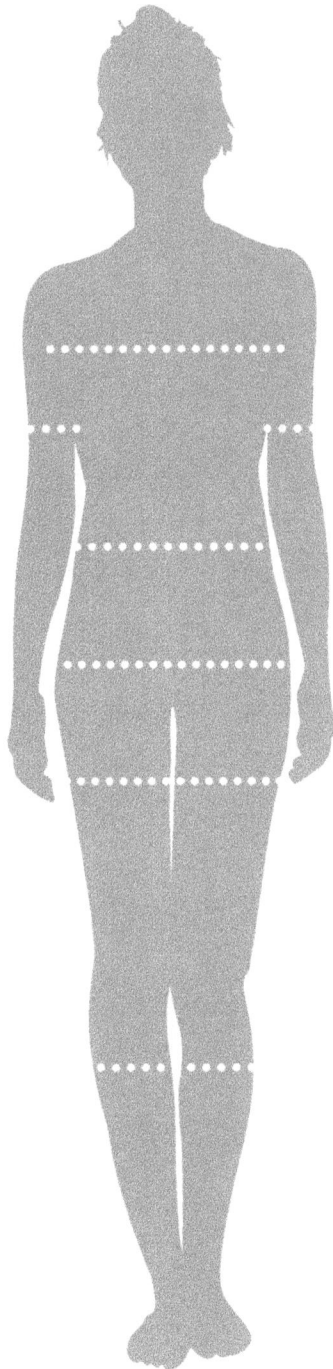

BEFORE

DATE

CHEST

LEFT ARM

RIGHT ARM

WAIST

HIPS

LEFT THIGH

RIGHT THIGH

LEFT CALF

RIGHT CALF

WEIGHT

NOTES

AFTER

DATE

CHEST

LEFT ARM

RIGHT ARM

WAIST

HIPS

LEFT THIGH

LEFT CALF

RIGHT CALF

WEIGHT

BODY MEASUREMENTS TRACKER

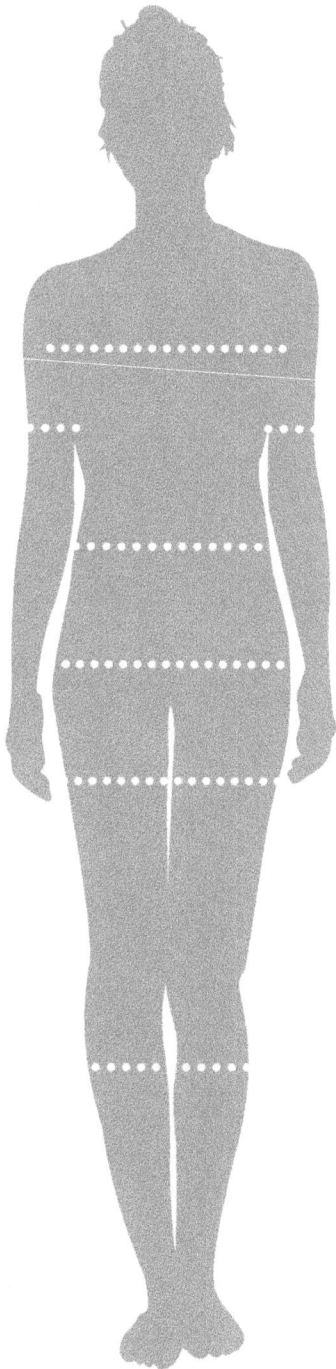

BEFORE

DATE

CHEST

LEFT ARM

RIGHT ARM

WAIST

HIPS

LEFT THIGH

RIGHT THIGH

LEFT CALF

RIGHT CALF

WEIGHT

NOTES

AFTER

DATE

CHEST

LEFT ARM

RIGHT ARM

WAIST

HIPS

LEFT THIGH

LEFT CALF

RIGHT CALF

WEIGHT

BODY MEASUREMENTS TRACKER

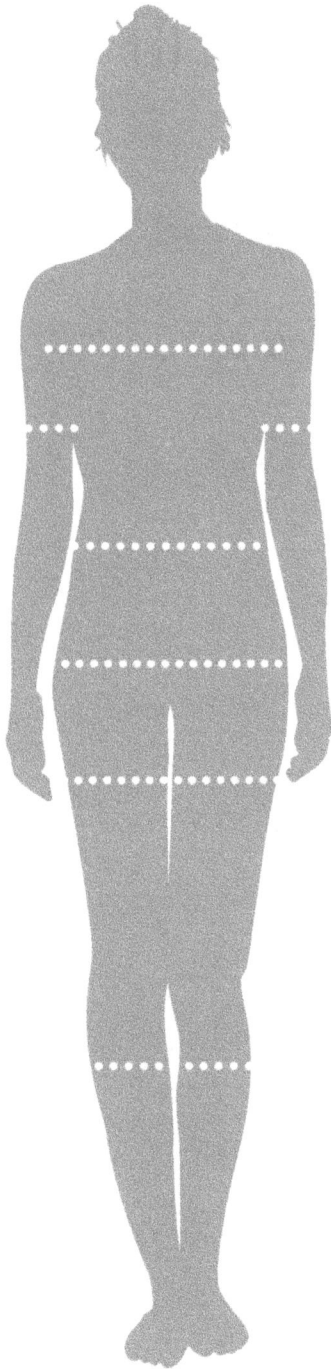

BEFORE

DATE

CHEST

LEFT ARM

RIGHT ARM

WAIST

HIPS

LEFT THIGH

RIGHT THIGH

LEFT CALF

RIGHT CALF

WEIGHT

NOTES

AFTER

DATE

CHEST

LEFT ARM

RIGHT ARM

WAIST

HIPS

LEFT THIGH

LEFT CALF

RIGHT CALF

WEIGHT

BODY MEASUREMENTS TRACKER

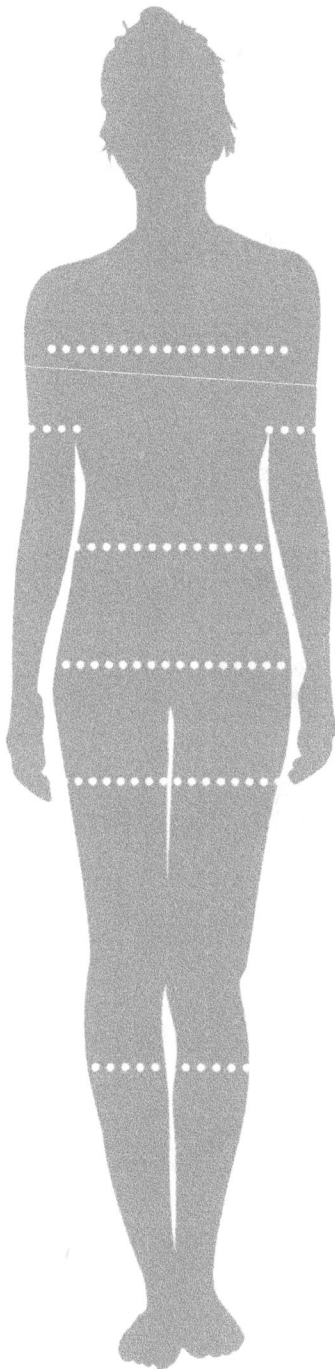

BEFORE

DATE

CHEST

LEFT ARM

RIGHT ARM

WAIST

HIPS

LEFT THIGH

RIGHT THIGH

LEFT CALF

RIGHT CALF

WEIGHT

NOTES

AFTER

DATE

CHEST

LEFT ARM

RIGHT ARM

WAIST

HIPS

LEFT THIGH

LEFT CALF

RIGHT CALF

WEIGHT

BODY MEASUREMENTS TRACKER

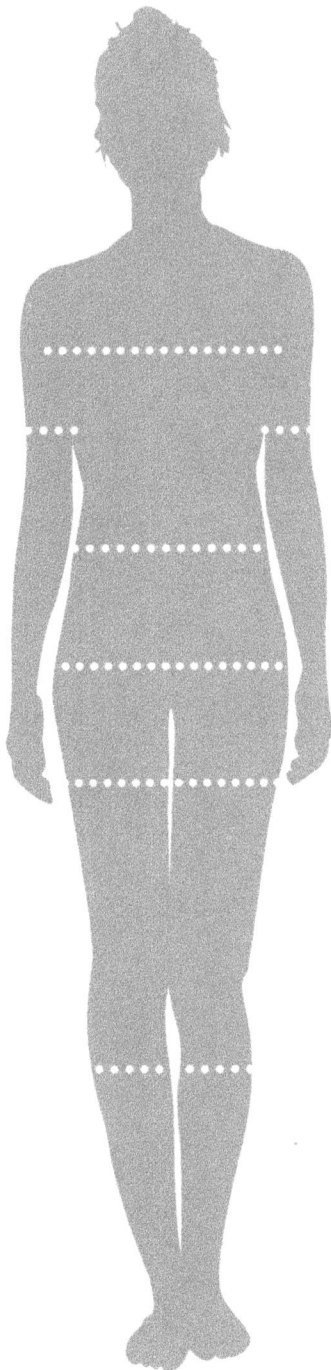

BEFORE

DATE

CHEST

LEFT ARM

RIGHT ARM

WAIST

HIPS

LEFT THIGH

RIGHT THIGH

LEFT CALF

RIGHT CALF

WEIGHT

NOTES

AFTER

DATE

CHEST

LEFT ARM

RIGHT ARM

WAIST

HIPS

LEFT THIGH

LEFT CALF

RIGHT CALF

WEIGHT

BODY MEASUREMENTS TRACKER

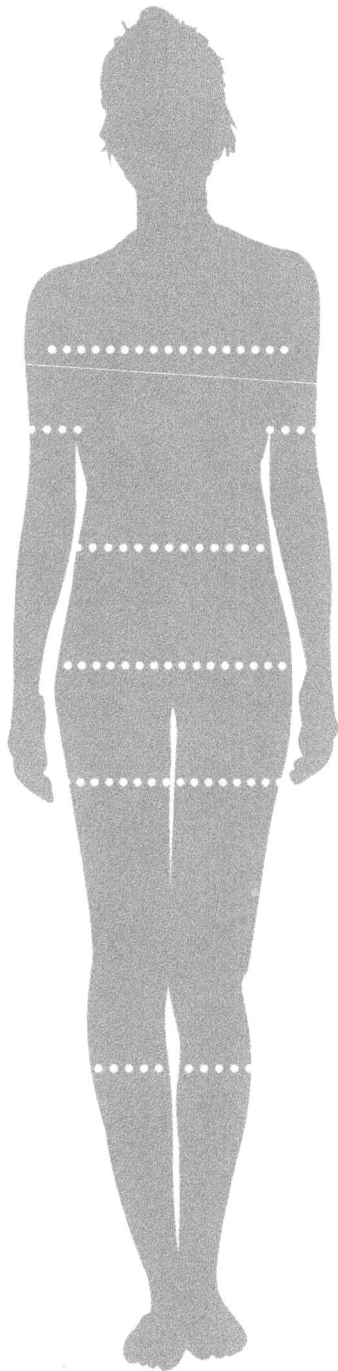

BEFORE	AFTER
DATE	DATE
CHEST	CHEST
LEFT ARM	LEFT ARM
RIGHT ARM	RIGHT ARM
WAIST	WAIST
HIPS	HIPS
LEFT THIGH	LEFT THIGH
RIGHT THIGH	RIGHT THIGH
LEFT CALF	LEFT CALF
RIGHT CALF	RIGHT CALF
WEIGHT	WEIGHT
NOTES	

BODY MEASUREMENTS TRACKER

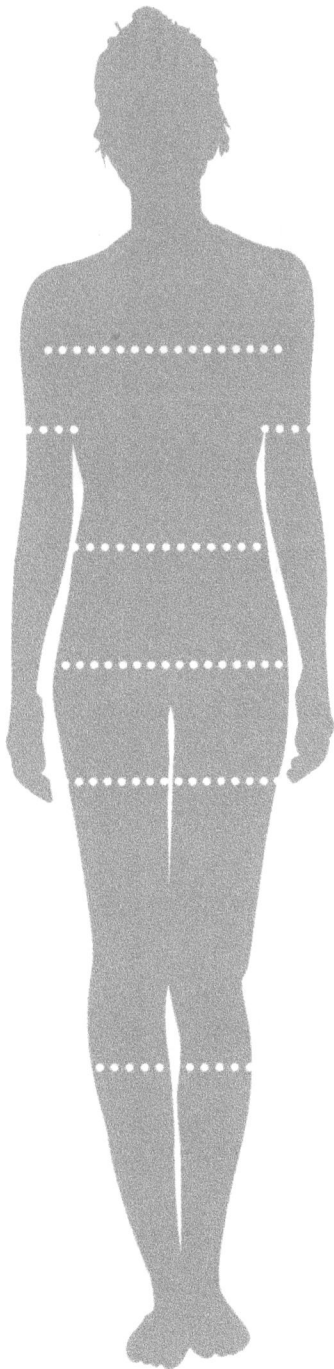

BEFORE

DATE

CHEST

LEFT ARM

RIGHT ARM

WAIST

HIPS

LEFT THIGH

RIGHT THIGH

LEFT CALF

RIGHT CALF

WEIGHT

NOTES

AFTER

DATE

CHEST

LEFT ARM

RIGHT ARM

WAIST

HIPS

LEFT THIGH

LEFT CALF

RIGHT CALF

WEIGHT

BODY MEASUREMENTS TRACKER

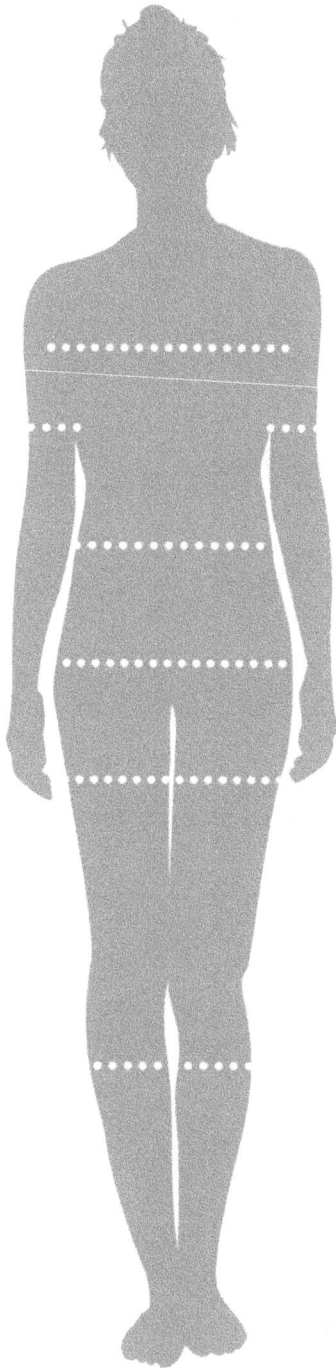

BEFORE

DATE

CHEST

LEFT ARM

RIGHT ARM

WAIST

HIPS

LEFT THIGH

RIGHT THIGH

LEFT CALF

RIGHT CALF

WEIGHT

NOTES

AFTER

DATE

CHEST

LEFT ARM

RIGHT ARM

WAIST

HIPS

LEFT THIGH

LEFT CALF

RIGHT CALF

WEIGHT

BODY MEASUREMENTS TRACKER

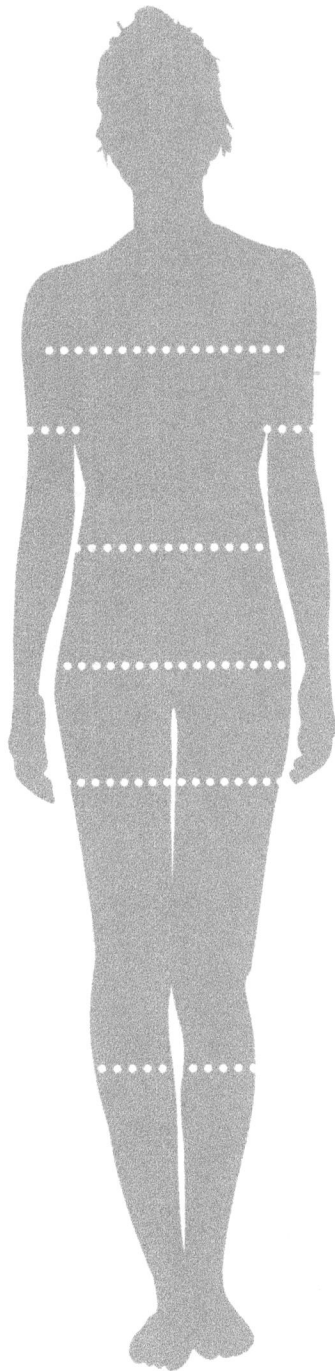

BEFORE

DATE

CHEST

LEFT ARM

RIGHT ARM

WAIST

HIPS

LEFT THIGH

RIGHT THIGH

LEFT CALF

RIGHT CALF

WEIGHT

NOTES

AFTER

DATE

CHEST

LEFT ARM

RIGHT ARM

WAIST

HIPS

LEFT THIGH

LEFT CALF

RIGHT CALF

WEIGHT

BODY MEASUREMENTS TRACKER

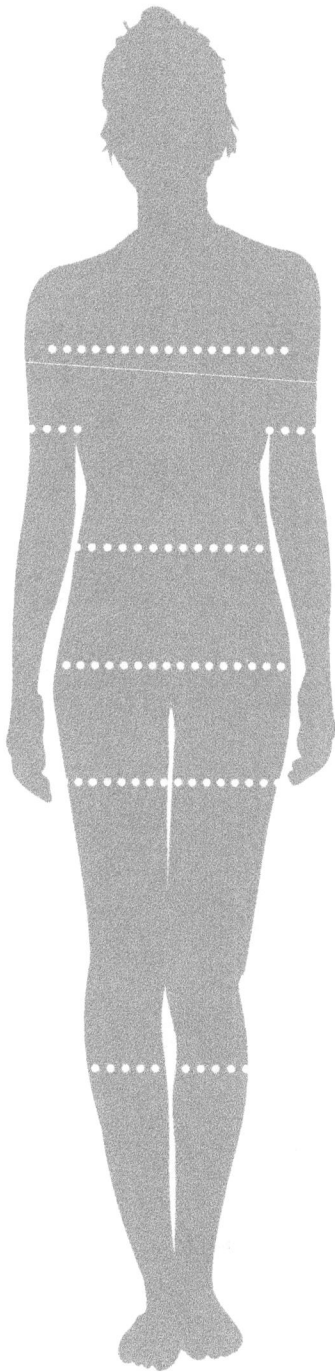

BEFORE

DATE

CHEST

LEFT ARM

RIGHT ARM

WAIST

HIPS

LEFT THIGH

RIGHT THIGH

LEFT CALF

RIGHT CALF

WEIGHT

NOTES

AFTER

DATE

CHEST

LEFT ARM

RIGHT ARM

WAIST

HIPS

LEFT THIGH

LEFT CALF

RIGHT CALF

WEIGHT

BODY MEASUREMENTS TRACKER

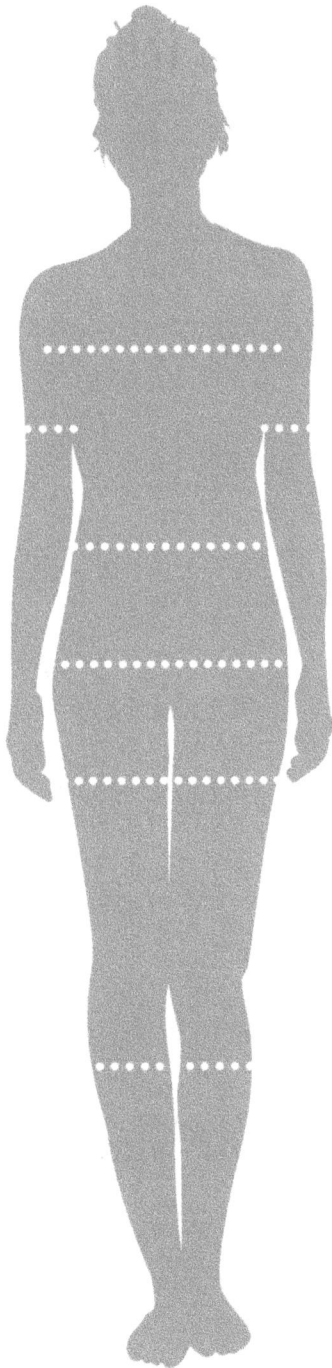

BEFORE

DATE

CHEST

LEFT ARM

RIGHT ARM

WAIST

HIPS

LEFT THIGH

RIGHT THIGH

LEFT CALF

RIGHT CALF

WEIGHT

NOTES

AFTER

DATE

CHEST

LEFT ARM

RIGHT ARM

WAIST

HIPS

LEFT THIGH

LEFT CALF

RIGHT CALF

WEIGHT

BODY MEASUREMENTS TRACKER

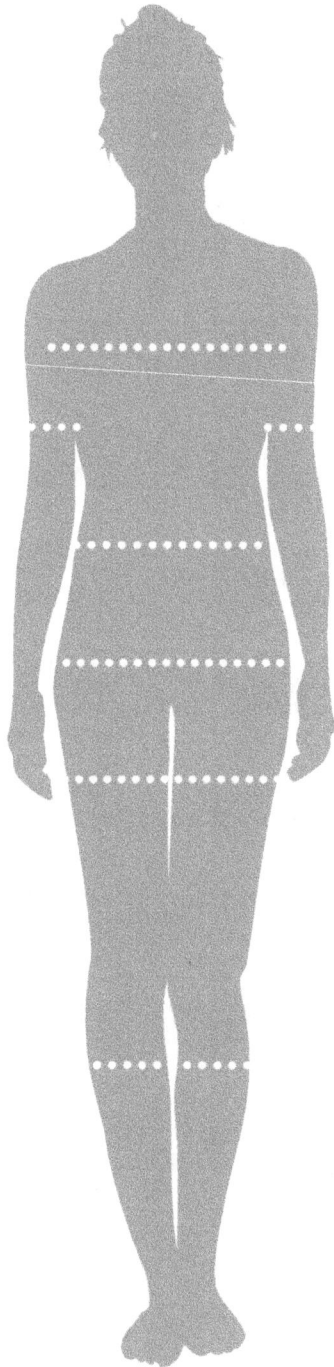

BEFORE

DATE

CHEST

LEFT ARM

RIGHT ARM

WAIST

HIPS

LEFT THIGH

RIGHT THIGH

LEFT CALF

RIGHT CALF

WEIGHT

NOTES

AFTER

DATE

CHEST

LEFT ARM

RIGHT ARM

WAIST

HIPS

LEFT THIGH

LEFT CALF

RIGHT CALF

WEIGHT

BODY MEASUREMENTS TRACKER

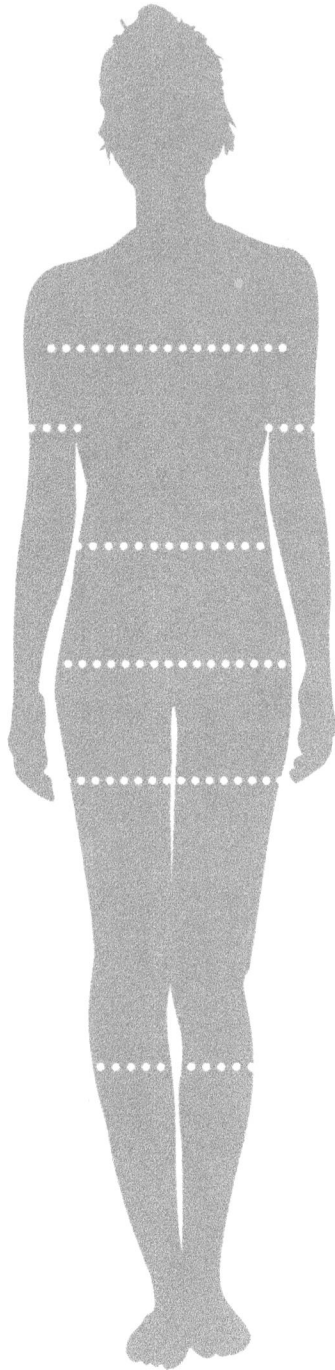

BEFORE

DATE

CHEST

LEFT ARM

RIGHT ARM

WAIST

HIPS

LEFT THIGH

RIGHT THIGH

LEFT CALF

RIGHT CALF

WEIGHT

NOTES

AFTER

DATE

CHEST

LEFT ARM

RIGHT ARM

WAIST

HIPS

LEFT THIGH

LEFT CALF

RIGHT CALF

WEIGHT

BODY MEASUREMENTS TRACKER

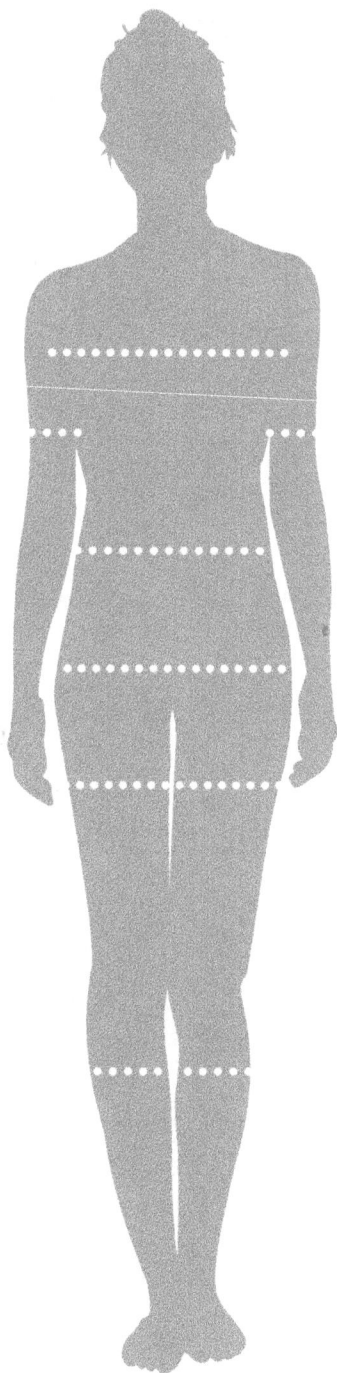

BEFORE

DATE

CHEST

LEFT ARM

RIGHT ARM

WAIST

HIPS

LEFT THIGH

RIGHT THIGH

LEFT CALF

RIGHT CALF

WEIGHT

NOTES

AFTER

DATE

CHEST

LEFT ARM

RIGHT ARM

WAIST

HIPS

LEFT THIGH

LEFT CALF

RIGHT CALF

WEIGHT

BODY MEASUREMENTS TRACKER

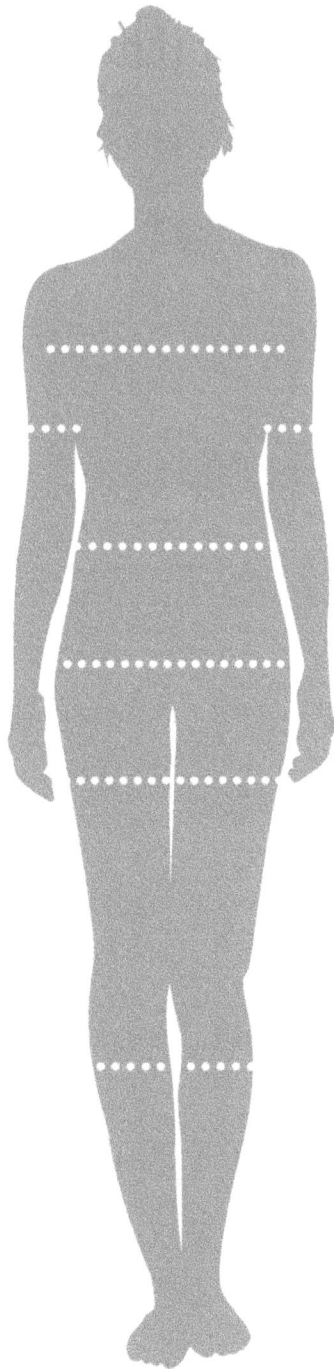

BEFORE

DATE

CHEST

LEFT ARM

RIGHT ARM

WAIST

HIPS

LEFT THIGH

RIGHT THIGH

LEFT CALF

RIGHT CALF

WEIGHT

NOTES

AFTER

DATE

CHEST

LEFT ARM

RIGHT ARM

WAIST

HIPS

LEFT THIGH

LEFT CALF

RIGHT CALF

WEIGHT

BODY MEASUREMENTS TRACKER

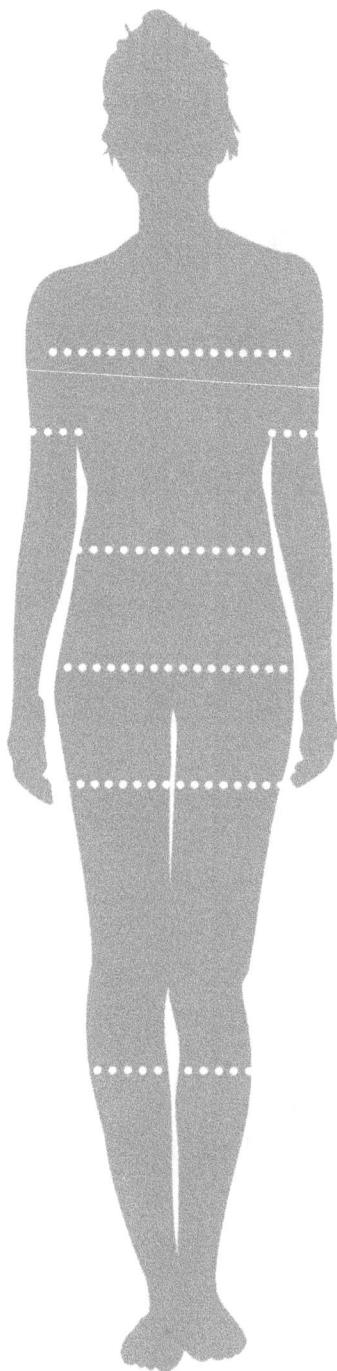

BEFORE

DATE

CHEST

LEFT ARM

RIGHT ARM

WAIST

HIPS

LEFT THIGH

RIGHT THIGH

LEFT CALF

RIGHT CALF

WEIGHT

NOTES

AFTER

DATE

CHEST

LEFT ARM

RIGHT ARM

WAIST

HIPS

LEFT THIGH

LEFT CALF

RIGHT CALF

WEIGHT

BODY MEASUREMENTS TRACKER

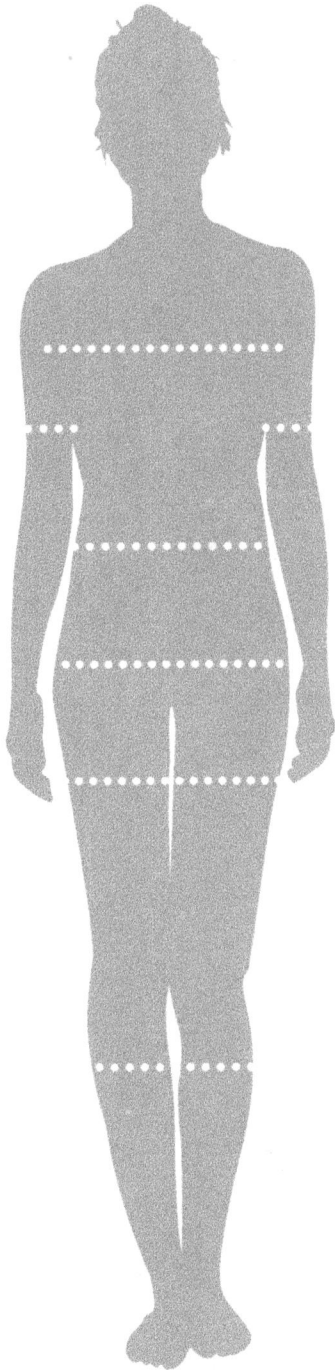

	BEFORE	AFTER
	DATE	DATE
	CHEST	CHEST
	LEFT ARM	LEFT ARM
	RIGHT ARM	RIGHT ARM
	WAIST	WAIST
	HIPS	HIPS
	LEFT THIGH	LEFT THIGH
	RIGHT THIGH	
	LEFT CALF	LEFT CALF
	RIGHT CALF	RIGHT CALF
	WEIGHT	WEIGHT

NOTES

BODY MEASUREMENTS TRACKER

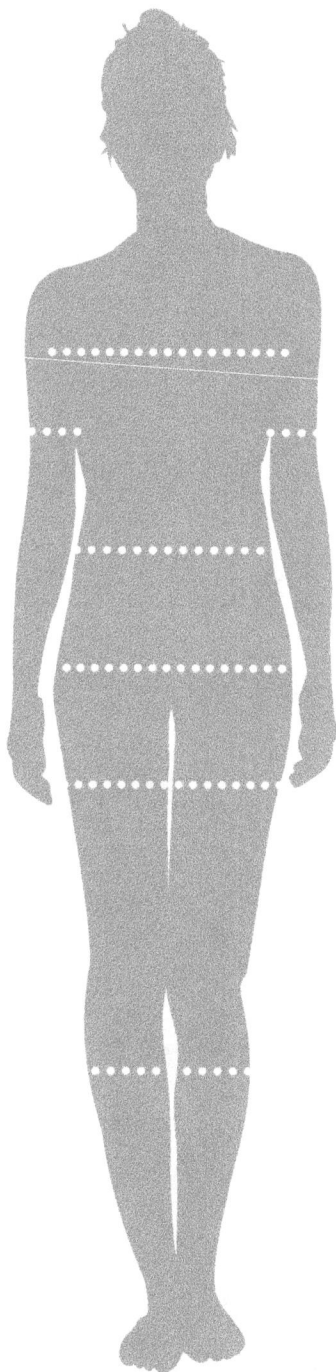

BEFORE

DATE	
CHEST	
LEFT ARM	
RIGHT ARM	
WAIST	
HIPS	
LEFT THIGH	
RIGHT THIGH	
LEFT CALF	
RIGHT CALF	
WEIGHT	

AFTER

DATE	
CHEST	
LEFT ARM	
RIGHT ARM	
WAIST	
HIPS	
LEFT THIGH	
LEFT CALF	
RIGHT CALF	
WEIGHT	

NOTES

BODY MEASUREMENTS TRACKER

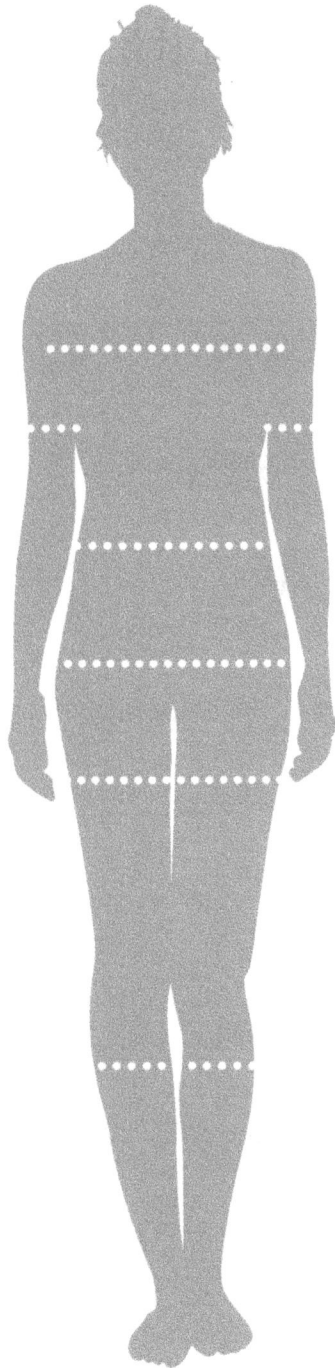

BEFORE

DATE

CHEST

LEFT ARM

RIGHT ARM

WAIST

HIPS

LEFT THIGH

RIGHT THIGH

LEFT CALF

RIGHT CALF

WEIGHT

NOTES

AFTER

DATE

CHEST

LEFT ARM

RIGHT ARM

WAIST

HIPS

LEFT THIGH

LEFT CALF

RIGHT CALF

WEIGHT

BODY MEASUREMENTS TRACKER

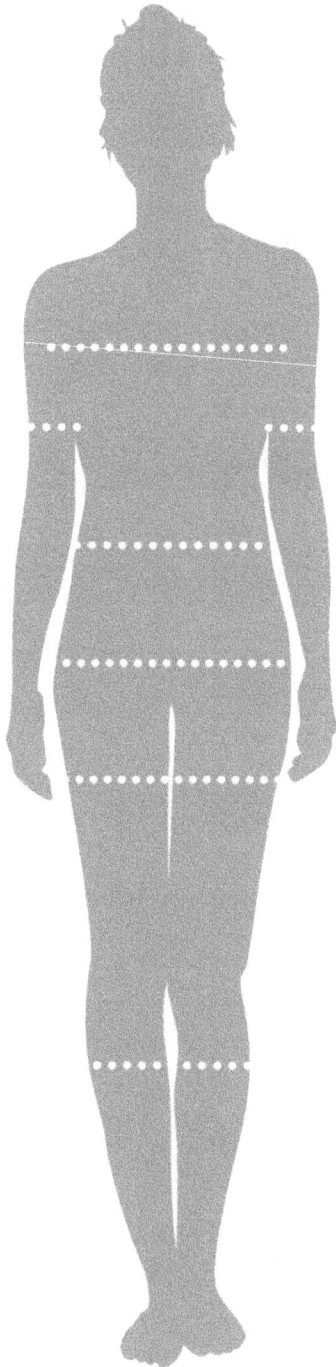

BEFORE

DATE

CHEST

LEFT ARM

RIGHT ARM

WAIST

HIPS

LEFT THIGH

RIGHT THIGH

LEFT CALF

RIGHT CALF

WEIGHT

NOTES

AFTER

DATE

CHEST

LEFT ARM

RIGHT ARM

WAIST

HIPS

LEFT THIGH

LEFT CALF

RIGHT CALF

WEIGHT

BODY MEASUREMENTS TRACKER

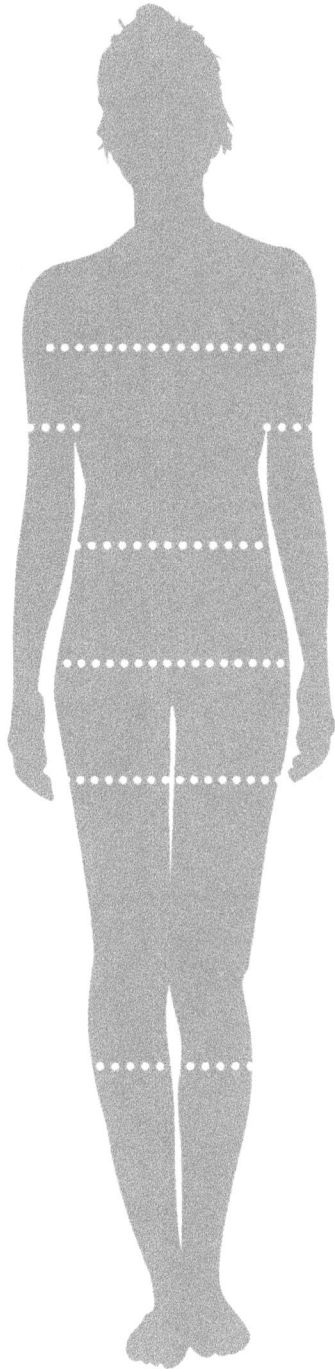

BEFORE

DATE	
CHEST	
LEFT ARM	
RIGHT ARM	
WAIST	
HIPS	
LEFT THIGH	
RIGHT THIGH	
LEFT CALF	
RIGHT CALF	
WEIGHT	

AFTER

DATE	
CHEST	
LEFT ARM	
RIGHT ARM	
WAIST	
HIPS	
LEFT THIGH	
LEFT CALF	
RIGHT CALF	
WEIGHT	

NOTES

BODY MEASUREMENTS TRACKER

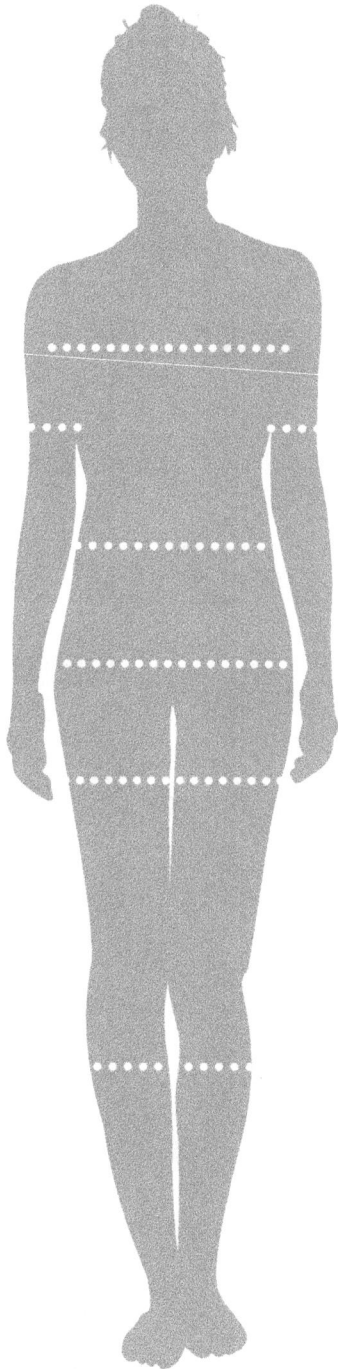

BEFORE

DATE

CHEST

LEFT ARM

RIGHT ARM

WAIST

HIPS

LEFT THIGH

RIGHT THIGH

LEFT CALF

RIGHT CALF

WEIGHT

NOTES

AFTER

DATE

CHEST

LEFT ARM

RIGHT ARM

WAIST

HIPS

LEFT THIGH

LEFT CALF

RIGHT CALF

WEIGHT

BODY MEASUREMENTS TRACKER

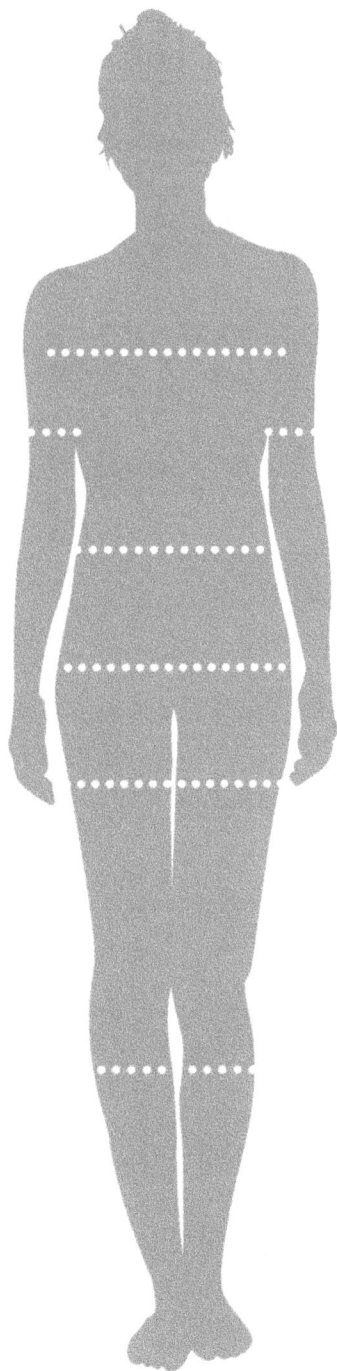

BEFORE

DATE	
CHEST	
LEFT ARM	
RIGHT ARM	
WAIST	
HIPS	
LEFT THIGH	
RIGHT THIGH	
LEFT CALF	
RIGHT CALF	
WEIGHT	
NOTES	

AFTER

DATE

CHEST

LEFT ARM

RIGHT ARM

WAIST

HIPS

LEFT THIGH

LEFT CALF

RIGHT CALF

WEIGHT

BODY MEASUREMENTS TRACKER

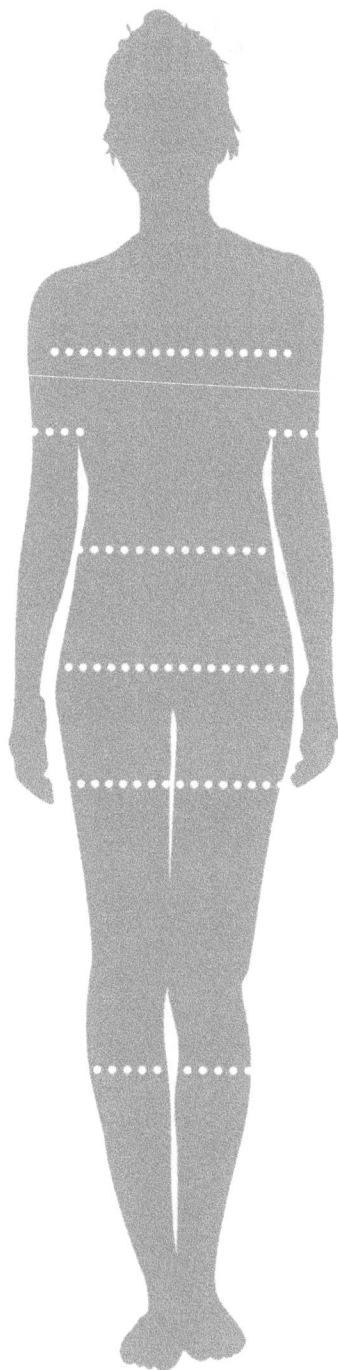

BEFORE

DATE

CHEST

LEFT ARM

RIGHT ARM

WAIST

HIPS

LEFT THIGH

RIGHT THIGH

LEFT CALF

RIGHT CALF

WEIGHT

NOTES

AFTER

DATE

CHEST

LEFT ARM

RIGHT ARM

WAIST

HIPS

LEFT THIGH

LEFT CALF

RIGHT CALF

WEIGHT

BODY MEASUREMENTS TRACKER

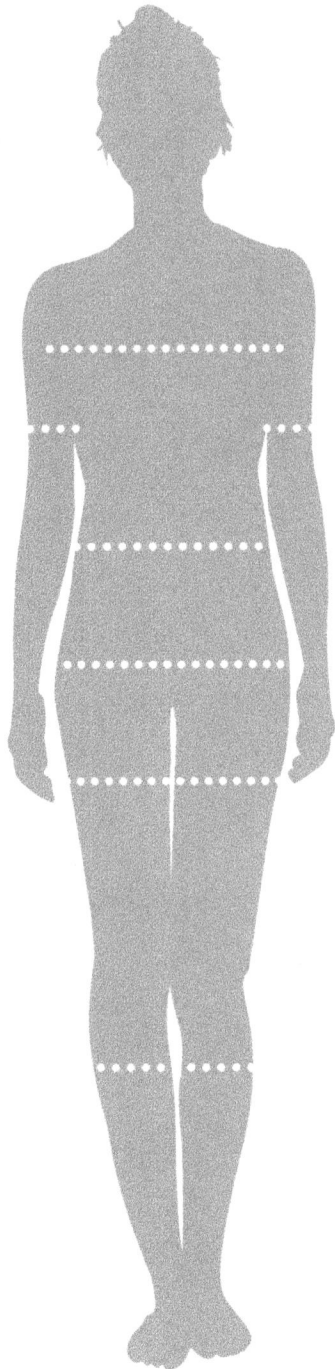

BEFORE

- DATE
- CHEST
- LEFT ARM
- RIGHT ARM
- WAIST
- HIPS
- LEFT THIGH
- RIGHT THIGH
- LEFT CALF
- RIGHT CALF
- WEIGHT

AFTER

- DATE
- CHEST
- LEFT ARM
- RIGHT ARM
- WAIST
- HIPS
- LEFT THIGH
- LEFT CALF
- RIGHT CALF
- WEIGHT

NOTES

BODY MEASUREMENTS TRACKER

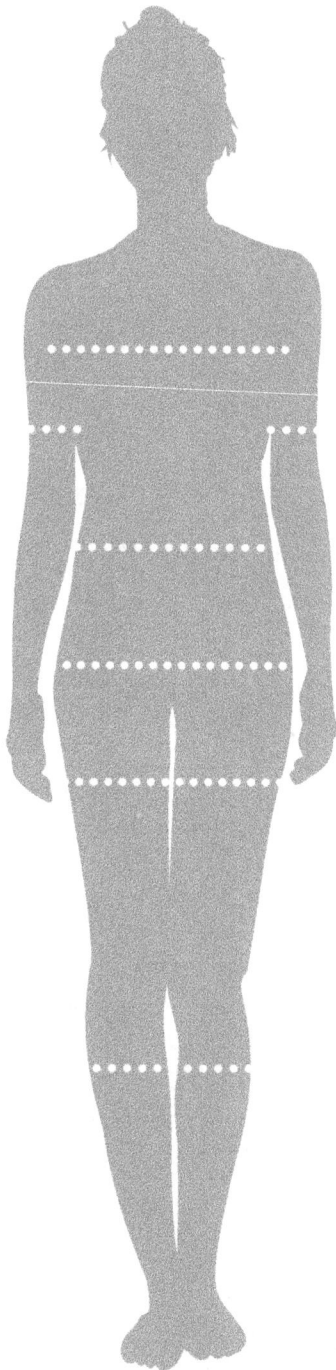

BEFORE

DATE

CHEST

LEFT ARM

RIGHT ARM

WAIST

HIPS

LEFT THIGH

RIGHT THIGH

LEFT CALF

RIGHT CALF

WEIGHT

NOTES

AFTER

DATE

CHEST

LEFT ARM

RIGHT ARM

WAIST

HIPS

LEFT THIGH

LEFT CALF

RIGHT CALF

WEIGHT

BODY MEASUREMENTS TRACKER

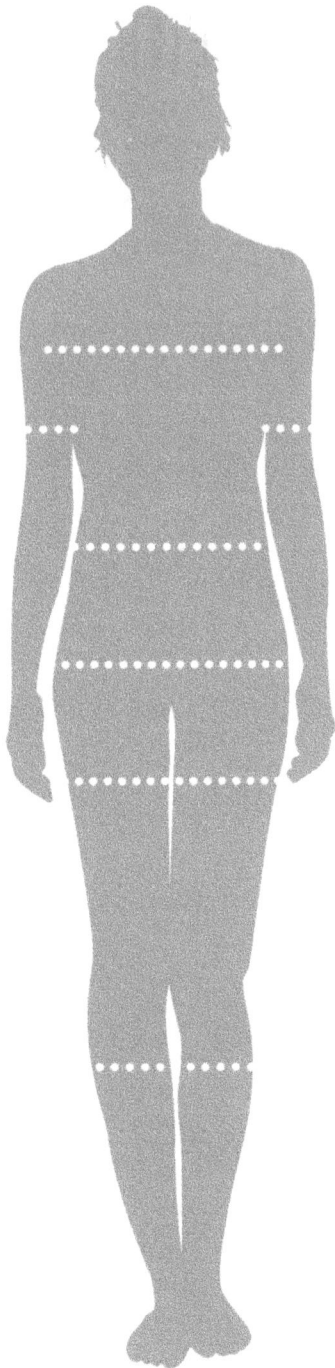

BEFORE	AFTER
DATE	DATE
CHEST	CHEST
LEFT ARM	LEFT ARM
RIGHT ARM	RIGHT ARM
WAIST	WAIST
HIPS	HIPS
LEFT THIGH	LEFT THIGH
RIGHT THIGH	
LEFT CALF	LEFT CALF
RIGHT CALF	RIGHT CALF
WEIGHT	WEIGHT
NOTES	

BODY MEASUREMENTS TRACKER

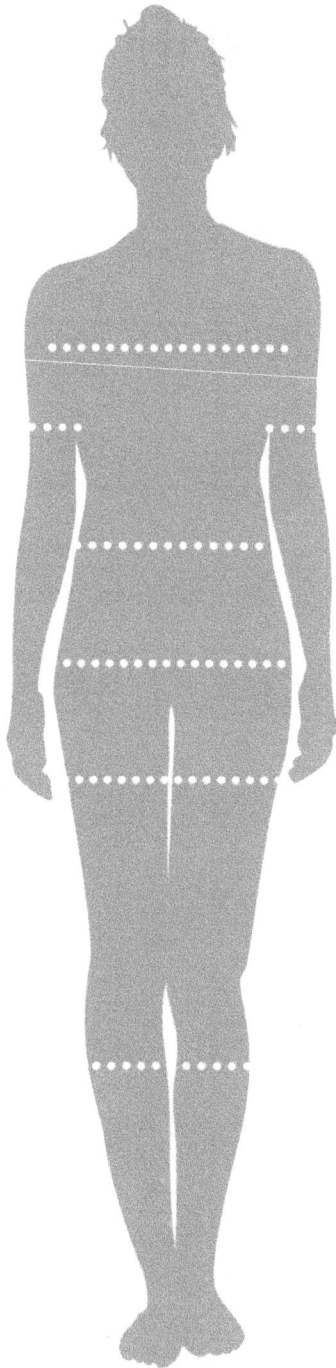

BEFORE

DATE

CHEST

LEFT ARM

RIGHT ARM

WAIST

HIPS

LEFT THIGH

RIGHT THIGH

LEFT CALF

RIGHT CALF

WEIGHT

NOTES

AFTER

DATE

CHEST

LEFT ARM

RIGHT ARM

WAIST

HIPS

LEFT THIGH

LEFT CALF

RIGHT CALF

WEIGHT

BODY MEASUREMENTS TRACKER

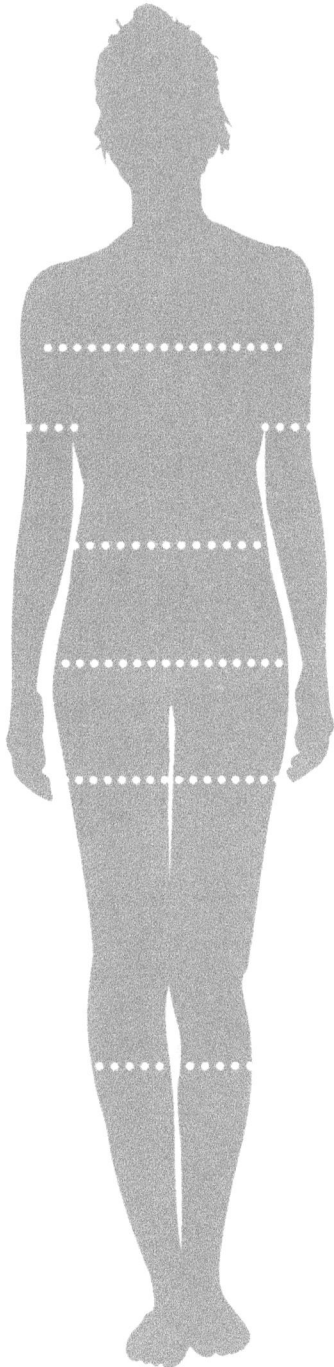

BEFORE

DATE

CHEST

LEFT ARM

RIGHT ARM

WAIST

HIPS

LEFT THIGH

RIGHT THIGH

LEFT CALF

RIGHT CALF

WEIGHT

NOTES

AFTER

DATE

CHEST

LEFT ARM

RIGHT ARM

WAIST

HIPS

LEFT THIGH

RIGHT THIGH

LEFT CALF

RIGHT CALF

WEIGHT

BODY MEASUREMENTS TRACKER

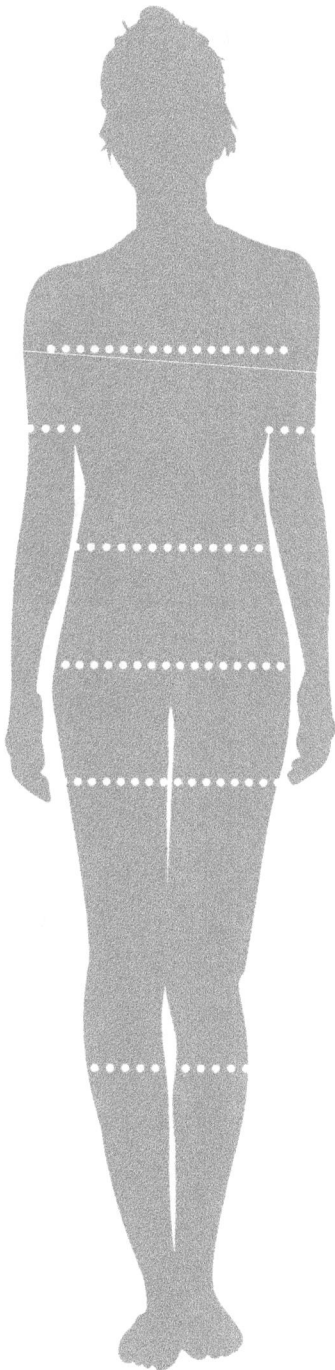

BEFORE

DATE

CHEST

LEFT ARM

RIGHT ARM

WAIST

HIPS

LEFT THIGH

RIGHT THIGH

LEFT CALF

RIGHT CALF

WEIGHT

NOTES

AFTER

DATE

CHEST

LEFT ARM

RIGHT ARM

WAIST

HIPS

LEFT THIGH

LEFT CALF

RIGHT CALF

WEIGHT

BODY MEASUREMENTS TRACKER

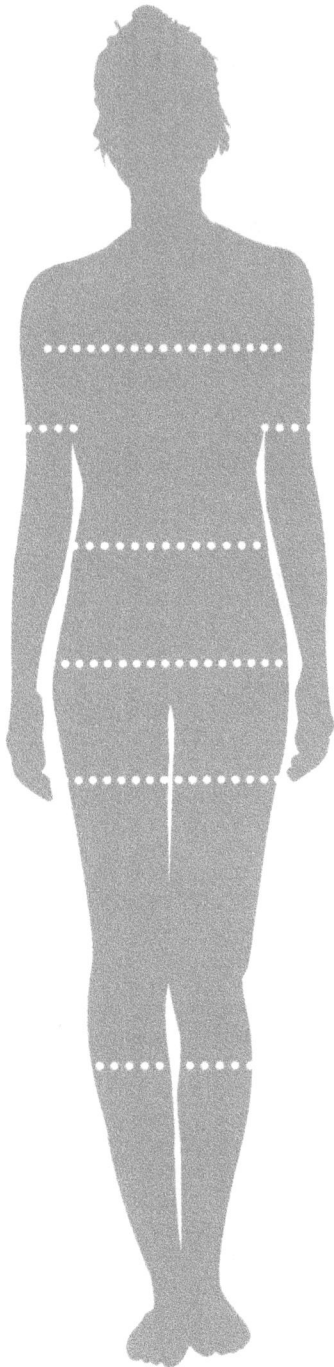

BEFORE

DATE

CHEST

LEFT ARM

RIGHT ARM

WAIST

HIPS

LEFT THIGH

RIGHT THIGH

LEFT CALF

RIGHT CALF

WEIGHT

NOTES

AFTER

DATE

CHEST

LEFT ARM

RIGHT ARM

WAIST

HIPS

LEFT THIGH

LEFT CALF

RIGHT CALF

WEIGHT

BODY MEASUREMENTS TRACKER

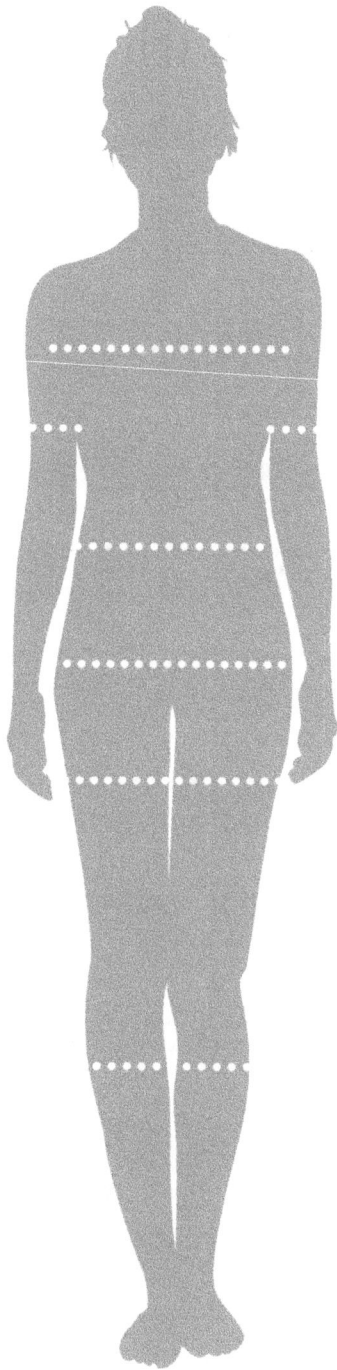

BEFORE

DATE

CHEST

LEFT ARM

RIGHT ARM

WAIST

HIPS

LEFT THIGH

RIGHT THIGH

LEFT CALF

RIGHT CALF

WEIGHT

NOTES

AFTER

DATE

CHEST

LEFT ARM

RIGHT ARM

WAIST

HIPS

LEFT THIGH

LEFT CALF

RIGHT CALF

WEIGHT

BODY MEASUREMENTS TRACKER

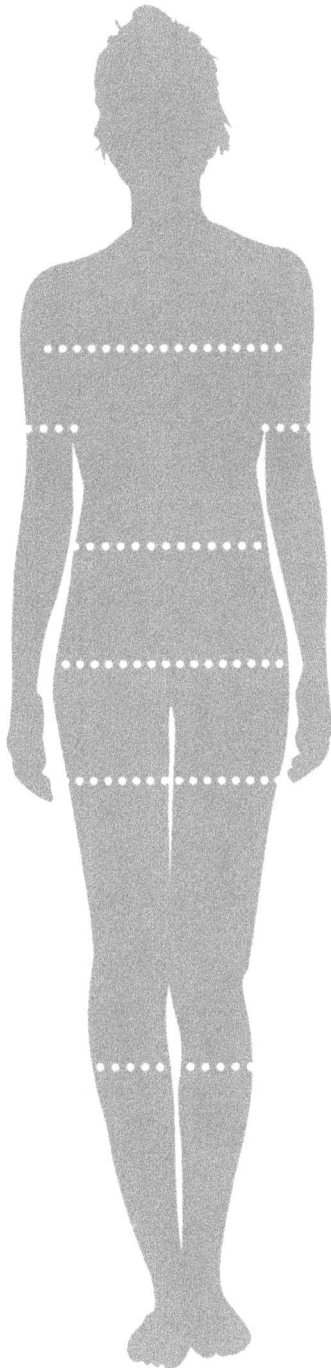

BEFORE

DATE	
CHEST	
LEFT ARM	
RIGHT ARM	
WAIST	
HIPS	
LEFT THIGH	
RIGHT THIGH	
LEFT CALF	
RIGHT CALF	
WEIGHT	

AFTER

DATE	
CHEST	
LEFT ARM	
RIGHT ARM	
WAIST	
HIPS	
LEFT THIGH	
LEFT CALF	
RIGHT CALF	
WEIGHT	

NOTES

BODY MEASUREMENTS TRACKER

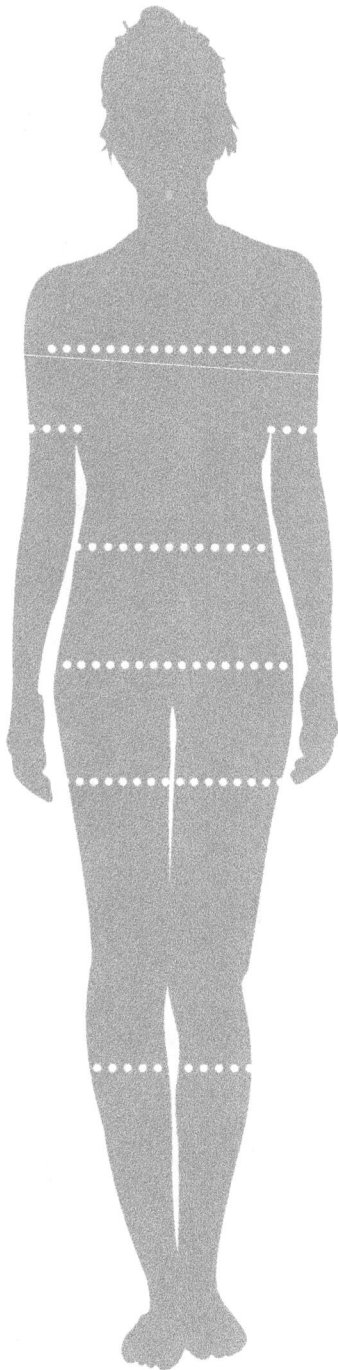

BEFORE

DATE

CHEST

LEFT ARM

RIGHT ARM

WAIST

HIPS

LEFT THIGH

RIGHT THIGH

LEFT CALF

RIGHT CALF

WEIGHT

NOTES

AFTER

DATE

CHEST

LEFT ARM

RIGHT ARM

WAIST

HIPS

LEFT THIGH

LEFT CALF

RIGHT CALF

WEIGHT

BODY MEASUREMENTS TRACKER

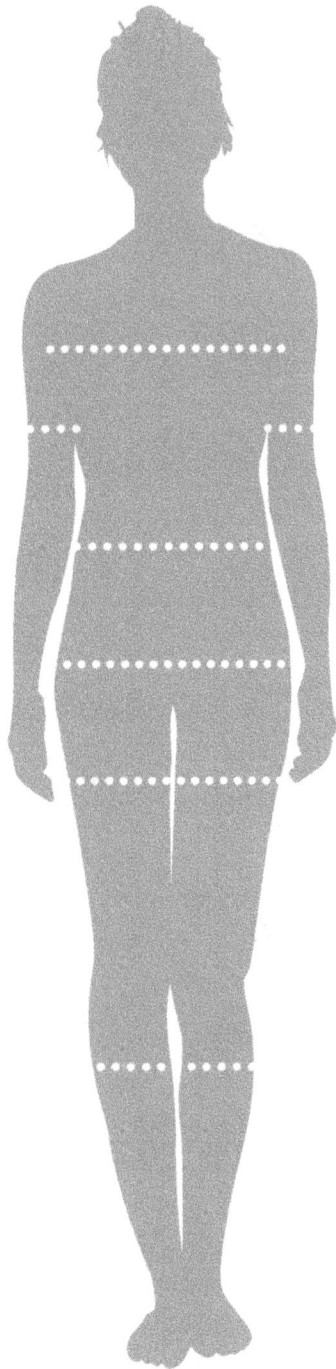

BEFORE

DATE

CHEST

LEFT ARM

RIGHT ARM

WAIST

HIPS

LEFT THIGH

RIGHT THIGH

LEFT CALF

RIGHT CALF

WEIGHT

NOTES

AFTER

DATE

CHEST

LEFT ARM

RIGHT ARM

WAIST

HIPS

LEFT THIGH

LEFT CALF

RIGHT CALF

WEIGHT

BODY MEASUREMENTS TRACKER

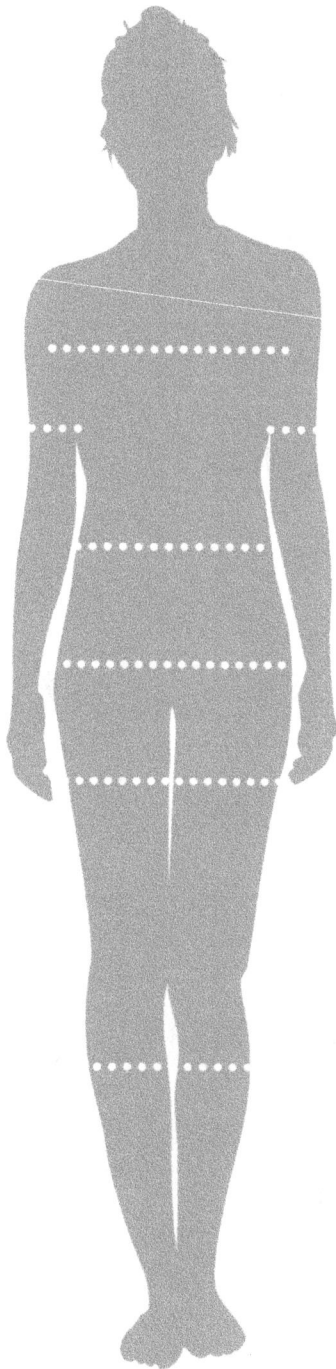

BEFORE

DATE

CHEST

LEFT ARM

RIGHT ARM

WAIST

HIPS

LEFT THIGH

RIGHT THIGH

LEFT CALF

RIGHT CALF

WEIGHT

NOTES

AFTER

DATE

CHEST

LEFT ARM

RIGHT ARM

WAIST

HIPS

LEFT THIGH

LEFT CALF

RIGHT CALF

WEIGHT

BODY MEASUREMENTS TRACKER

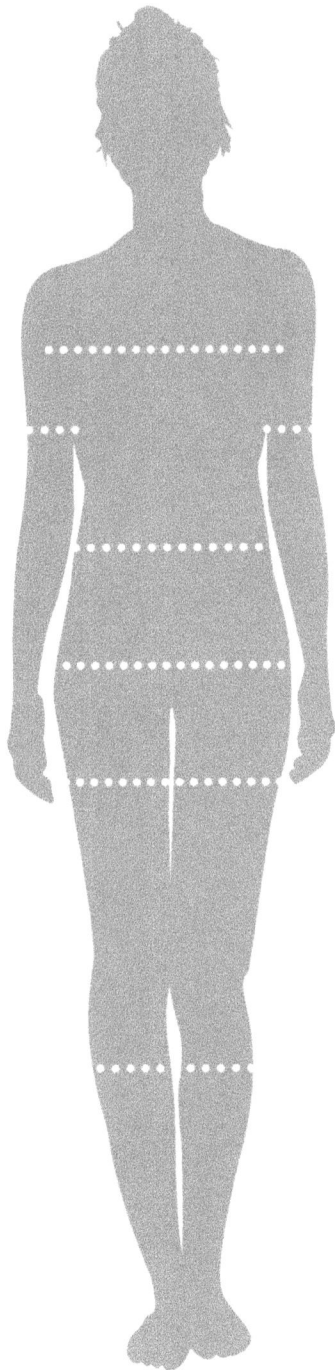

BEFORE

DATE

CHEST

LEFT ARM

RIGHT ARM

WAIST

HIPS

LEFT THIGH

RIGHT THIGH

LEFT CALF

RIGHT CALF

WEIGHT

NOTES

AFTER

DATE

CHEST

LEFT ARM

RIGHT ARM

WAIST

HIPS

LEFT THIGH

LEFT CALF

RIGHT CALF

WEIGHT

BODY MEASUREMENTS TRACKER

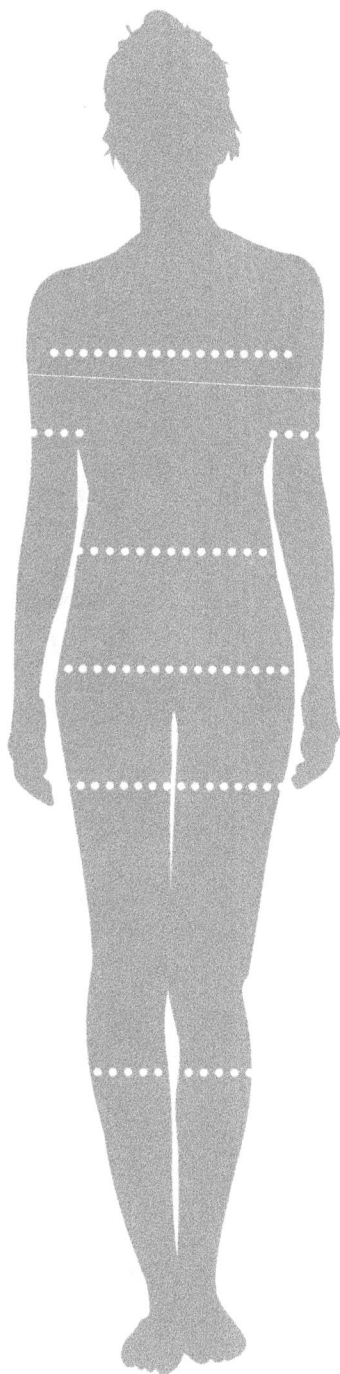

BEFORE

DATE

CHEST

LEFT ARM

RIGHT ARM

WAIST

HIPS

LEFT THIGH

RIGHT THIGH

LEFT CALF

RIGHT CALF

WEIGHT

NOTES

AFTER

DATE

CHEST

LEFT ARM

RIGHT ARM

WAIST

HIPS

LEFT THIGH

LEFT CALF

RIGHT CALF

WEIGHT

BODY MEASUREMENTS TRACKER

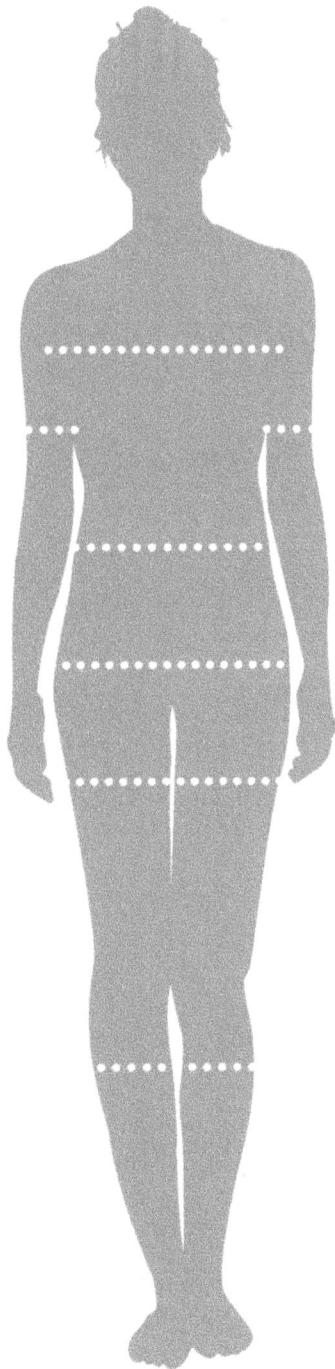

BEFORE

DATE

CHEST

LEFT ARM

RIGHT ARM

WAIST

HIPS

LEFT THIGH

RIGHT THIGH

LEFT CALF

RIGHT CALF

WEIGHT

NOTES

AFTER

DATE

CHEST

LEFT ARM

RIGHT ARM

WAIST

HIPS

LEFT THIGH

LEFT CALF

RIGHT CALF

WEIGHT

BODY MEASUREMENTS TRACKER

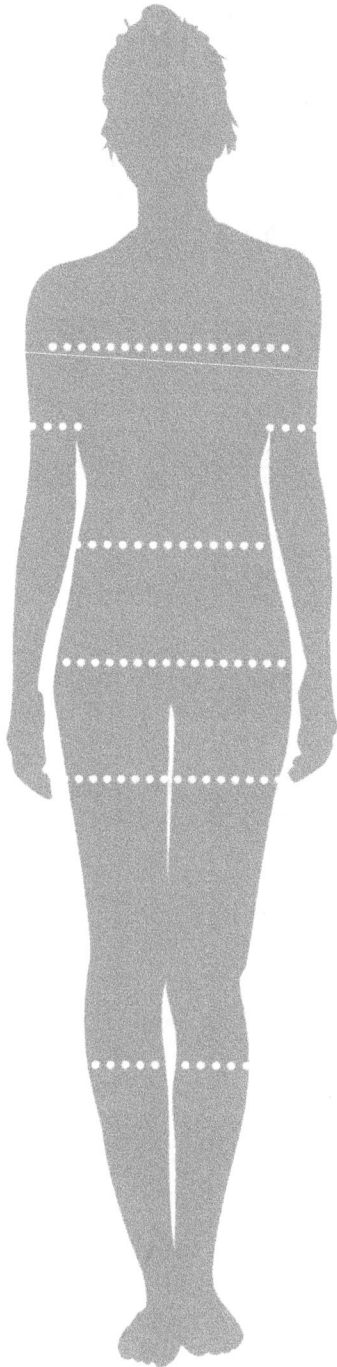

BEFORE

DATE

CHEST

LEFT ARM

RIGHT ARM

WAIST

HIPS

LEFT THIGH

RIGHT THIGH

LEFT CALF

RIGHT CALF

WEIGHT

NOTES

AFTER

DATE

CHEST

LEFT ARM

RIGHT ARM

WAIST

HIPS

LEFT THIGH

LEFT CALF

RIGHT CALF

WEIGHT

BODY MEASUREMENTS TRACKER

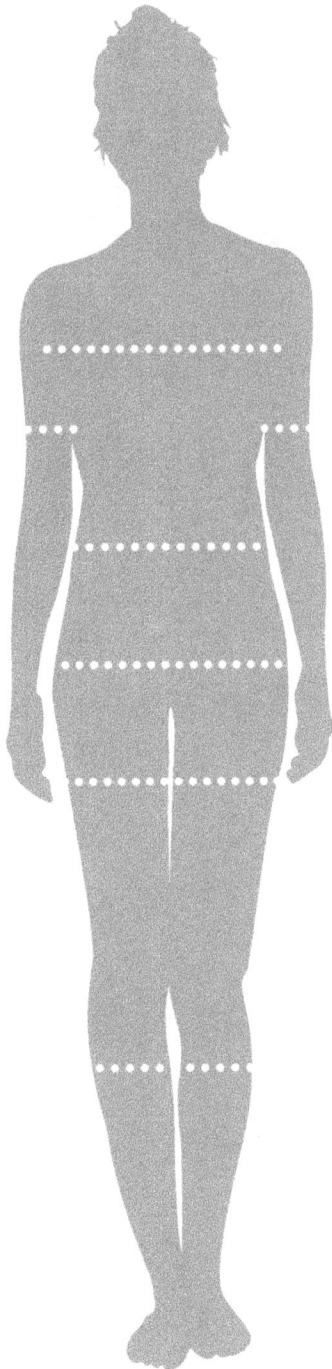

BEFORE	AFTER
DATE	DATE
CHEST	CHEST
LEFT ARM	LEFT ARM
RIGHT ARM	RIGHT ARM
WAIST	WAIST
HIPS	HIPS
LEFT THIGH	LEFT THIGH
RIGHT THIGH	
LEFT CALF	LEFT CALF
RIGHT CALF	RIGHT CALF
WEIGHT	WEIGHT
NOTES	

BODY MEASUREMENTS TRACKER

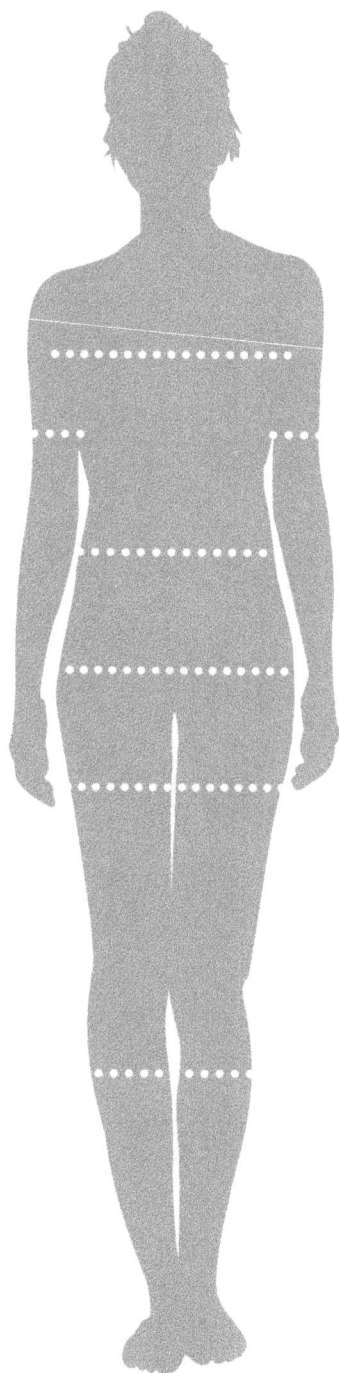

BEFORE

DATE	
CHEST	
LEFT ARM	
RIGHT ARM	
WAIST	
HIPS	
LEFT THIGH	
RIGHT THIGH	
LEFT CALF	
RIGHT CALF	
WEIGHT	

NOTES

AFTER

DATE	
CHEST	
LEFT ARM	
RIGHT ARM	
WAIST	
HIPS	
LEFT THIGH	
LEFT CALF	
RIGHT CALF	
WEIGHT	

BODY MEASUREMENTS TRACKER

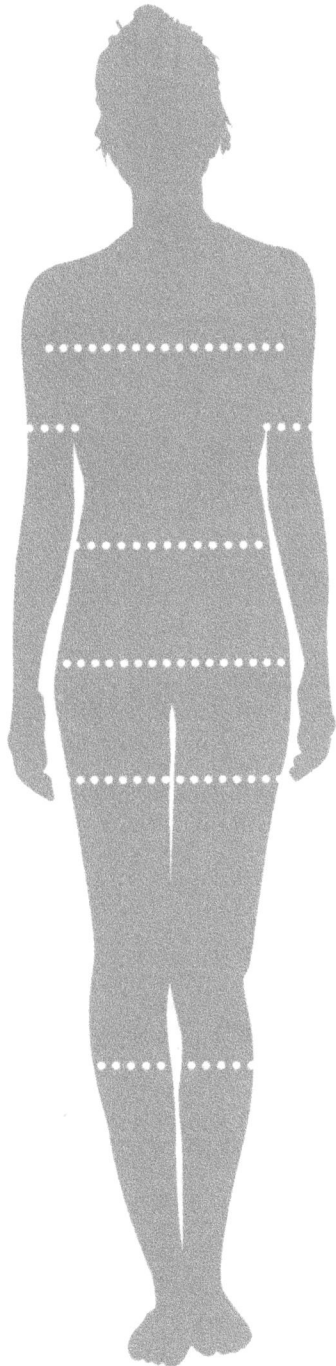

BEFORE

DATE

CHEST

LEFT ARM

RIGHT ARM

WAIST

HIPS

LEFT THIGH

RIGHT THIGH

LEFT CALF

RIGHT CALF

WEIGHT

NOTES

AFTER

DATE

CHEST

LEFT ARM

RIGHT ARM

WAIST

HIPS

LEFT THIGH

LEFT CALF

RIGHT CALF

WEIGHT

BODY MEASUREMENTS TRACKER

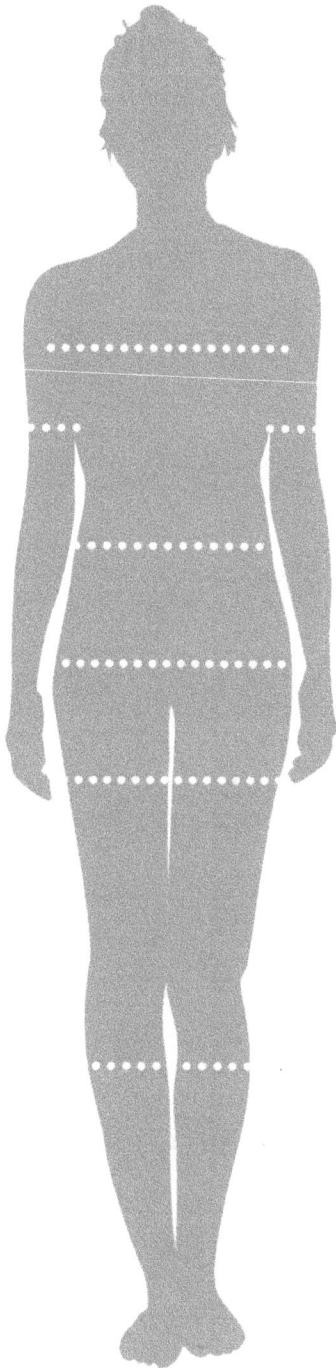

BEFORE

DATE

CHEST

LEFT ARM

RIGHT ARM

WAIST

HIPS

LEFT THIGH

RIGHT THIGH

LEFT CALF

RIGHT CALF

WEIGHT

NOTES

AFTER

DATE

CHEST

LEFT ARM

RIGHT ARM

WAIST

HIPS

LEFT THIGH

LEFT CALF

RIGHT CALF

WEIGHT

BODY MEASUREMENTS TRACKER

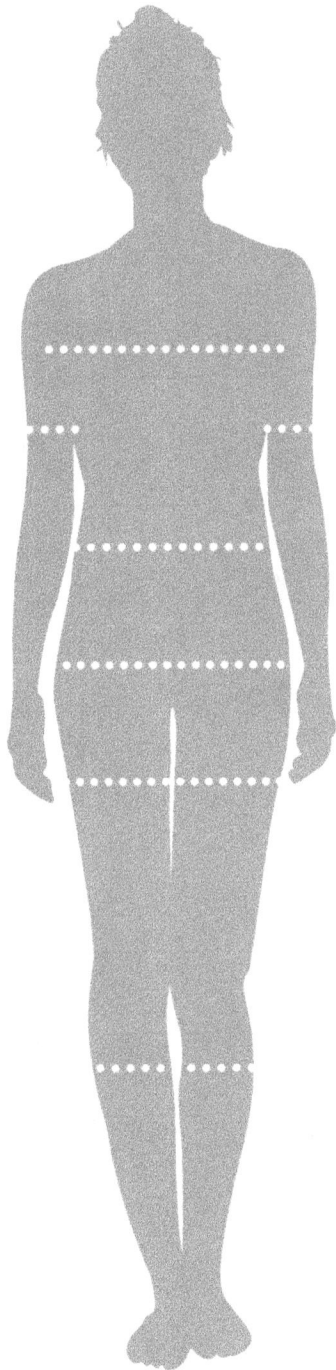

BEFORE

DATE

CHEST

LEFT ARM

RIGHT ARM

WAIST

HIPS

LEFT THIGH

RIGHT THIGH

LEFT CALF

RIGHT CALF

WEIGHT

NOTES

AFTER

DATE

CHEST

LEFT ARM

RIGHT ARM

WAIST

HIPS

LEFT THIGH

LEFT CALF

RIGHT CALF

WEIGHT

BODY MEASUREMENTS TRACKER

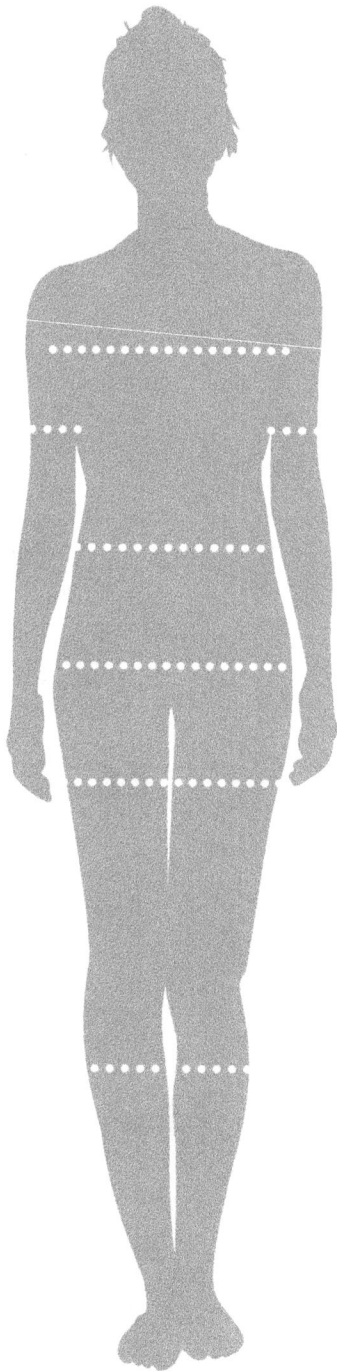

	BEFORE	AFTER
DATE		
CHEST		
LEFT ARM		
RIGHT ARM		
WAIST		
HIPS		
LEFT THIGH		
RIGHT THIGH		
LEFT CALF		
RIGHT CALF		
WEIGHT		

NOTES

BODY MEASUREMENTS TRACKER

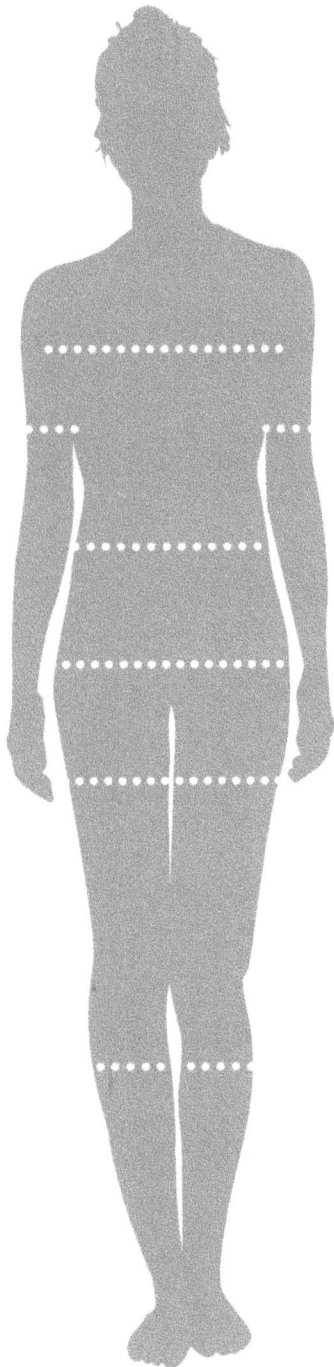

BEFORE

DATE

CHEST

LEFT ARM

RIGHT ARM

WAIST

HIPS

LEFT THIGH

RIGHT THIGH

LEFT CALF

RIGHT CALF

WEIGHT

NOTES

AFTER

DATE

CHEST

LEFT ARM

RIGHT ARM

WAIST

HIPS

LEFT THIGH

LEFT CALF

RIGHT CALF

WEIGHT

www.ingramcontent.com/pod-product-compliance
Lightning Source LLC
Chambersburg PA
CBHW080559030426

42336CB00019B/3256